FIXING
YOUR FEET

Prevention and Treatments
for Athletes

Second Edition

"This is a book for people who want common sense treatments for foot problems, not classroom or clinic theories of little value."
David Hannaford, DPM, Sports Podiatrist to many Olympians, ultramarthoners, adventure racers, and other endurance athletes.

*"All too often the real source of a knee, hip, or back injury is overlooked because people forget the foot is more than just a means of getting from point "A" to point "B". The foot is the beginning of the body's contact with the earth, a point of communion where the forces from the soil are absorbed and lessened. When the foot fails its mission, the whole body suffers. For an athlete, this is where a successful walk in the park or a winning marathon begins: at man's most under-appreciated appendage. **Fixing Your Feet** does a wonderful job of finally giving us a book dedicated to feet. Every active person should have it in his or her personal library."*
Jay Hodde, Certified Athletic Trainer, MS, ATC/L

*"I found immediate results in reducing and eliminating foot problems associated with multi-day adventure racing by following the steps outlined in **Fixing Your Feet**. Knowing how to take care of your feet may be the single most important factor in finishing an adventure race. This work and compilation of research on foot care is integral to the growth of adventure racing since foot problems are the number one reason most people do not finish the longer races. **Fixing Your Feet's** expertise translates hard learned lessons into sound practical advice that will only enhance your athletic performance and fills the void of information on this very vital topic. If you are ready to shorten your learning curve and concentrate on other aspects of the sport, I highly recommend that you read this book."*
Don Mann, Odyssey Adventure Racing Academy

"This is a complete and practical synopsis on proper foot care and can be used as a reference for almost any problem that runners or hikers may encounter."
Norman Klein, Race Director of the Sunmart Texas Trail Runs and former race director of the Western States 100 Mile Endurance Run.

*"Get a toehold on the blister situation before they cost you a finish. **Fixing Your Feet** should be read before any multi-day event. Definitely a 'two toes up'!"*
Cathy Tibbetts, Ultrarunner and Adventure Racer

"The best, most readable, practical and useful book on foot care that I've ever seen."
George Beinhorn. Ultrarunner

FIXING YOUR FEET

Prevention and Treatments for Athletes

Second Edition

John Vonhof

Footwork **FP** Publications
Fremont, CA 94536
www.footworkpub.com

Cover design copyright © 2000 by Kozak Design
Cover illustration copyright © 1997 by Adam Caldwell
Cover photographs copyright © 1997, Dan Campbell Photography, Gay Wiseman, and John Vonhof
Illustrations copyright © 2000 by John Vonhof

ISBN: 0-9657386-0-4
Library of Congress Catalog Card Number: 00-190112

FIXING YOUR FEET: Prevention and Treatments for Athletes. Second edition. Copyright © 2000 by John Vonhof. Published by Footwork Publications, 4438 Gibraltar Drive, Fremont, CA 94536. Printed in the United States of America by KNI, Inc.

Dedication

The second edition of *Fixing Your Feet* is dedicated to the athletes who are training and racing in their sport, and stressing their feet, often to the extreme. As they train and race, their feet hurt and the ideas and tips in this book become important to them. They are the reason for this book.

I thank my wife, Kathie, for her continued patience through the rewrite and research process and to my son, Scott, who after one of my 12-hour track runs, had the idea for this book which became a reality in its first edition.

The book is also dedicated to the memory of my friend and ultrarunner, Dick Collins. Those of us who knew Dick will never forget him. Dick was the epitome of what our sport needs: he was a good listener—always ready with encouragement, he was warm and sincere—taking honest pleasure in your success, and he was always ready to lend a hand where needed—believing we should get involved in supporting and promoting our sports. He would have supported this book, because it follows his values in helping others.

Acknowledgements

A special thanks to all the athletes who have contributed their ideas on footcare that they learned through trial and error.

Thanks to Rich Schick, Physician's Assistant and ultrarunner, for reviewing the first edition and making many helpful suggestions on content.

Thanks to Dr. Bill Trolan, an emergency room physician, medical consultant to adventure racing teams, adventure racer, runner, hiker, and climber, for reviewing the first edition manuscript and providing his expertise and medical perspectives.

Thanks to Dennis Grandy, D.P.M. and David Hannaford, D.P.M. who reviewed the first edition manuscript and provided valuable insights and advice from their podiatrist's perspective.

Thanks to Kirk Boisseree and Karl King for reviewing the first edition manuscript.

Thanks to Gary Cantrell and Suzi Thibeault (foot taping techniques), Andrew Lovy (lubricants), and Tom Crawford (skin tougheners), for their willingness to share what they have learned about how these factors affect foot care.

Thanks to *Ultrarunning* magazine for permission to reprint portions of Gary Cantrell's article, "From the South: The Amazing Miracle of Duct Tape," and Andrew Lovy's article, "New Blister Formula Revealed! Free!"

Foreword – Second Edition

As I was limping over the last sand dune on the last day of the 7-day Marathon des Sables in the Moroccan Sahara desert, I thought of John Vonhof. I thought of his advice about foot protection. I was losing a toenail which could have been avoided had I heeded his advice about larger shoes in extreme heat. I thought I knew better. After all I have two silver buckles from the Western States 100-Mile Endurance Run, and being an experienced Sports Podiatrist I already fit my shoes roomy. But, as I looked around me, my little injury paled in comparison to the hundreds of runners limping to the finish with feet much more damaged than mine. Most of these foot problems could have been avoided with proper care.

John has not run this race, but he knows the proper preparation and foot care needed. He has become a scholar of extreme sport foot care. He has learned his subject in the trenches as a participant and as a volunteer at countless events. His own medical background gives him objectivity and hundreds of interviews add to his own written information base.

This book provides valuable insight into prevention, treatment, and understanding of the type of foot injuries encountered during hard activity. It is laced with practical pearls they don't teach in medical school. A beginner should use this book as a source for understanding fundamental prevention and care, but it also includes up to date methods and treatments that even the most experienced athlete needs.

So whether your interest is preventing friction in your first pair of racing flats or avoiding serious infection on your fifth day of a tropical adventure race this book has the answers. I know one person for sure who will read it again before he heads back to the Sahara ...me.

David Hannaford, DPM
Sports Podiatrist to many Olympians, runners and ultramarthoners, adventure racers, and other endurance athletes.

Foreword – First Edition

Ever since our first ancestors stepped on the ground, we have been plagued by foot problems, especially blisters. Now they continue to afflict us in a variety of ways. You see them on hikers, runners, and athletic pursuits of all manner and description.

The last few years have seen the beginnings of adventure racing. I am fortunate to have been a part of this exciting new development in outdoor activity. The one factor that continues to amaze me is that individuals and teams will spend vast amounts of money, time, and thought on training, equipment, and travel, but little or no preparation on their feet. Too often the result has been that within a few hours to a few days all that work has been ruined. Ruined because the primary mode of transportation has broken down with blisters.

This problem is universal with hikers, runners, and any activity that requires feet. Most of these problems could easily be avoided with some preventative care. Other foot problems could have been taken care of with early treatment, stopping a small problem from becoming a costly one.

This book is the result of two years of research and writing. John has combed through hundreds of articles and reviewed previous literature on foot care. He has interviewed a multitude of people, many of them athletes who push the envelope of human endurance and passed their knowledge on to you. Further, he has reviewed hundreds of products all connected to preventing foot and blister problems. This wealth of information has been distilled down to this most comprehensive and extremely well written book.

This is it—the best book ever written on foot care! Everyone who has been bothered by foot problems or wants to prevent them should own this book. Its encyclopedic knowledge never ceases to amaze me. Despite having spent four years reading and taking care of blisters and other foot problems, every time I open this book I gain new information.

Billy Trolan, MD
Emergency Room Physician, author of the *Blister Fighter Guide,* and medical consultant to adventure racing teams.

Contents

Introduction 1

Part One: The Basics

1. Seeking Medical Treatment 9
2. Sports and Your Feet 13
3. Conditioning 17
4. Biomechanics 19
5. Where You Run and Hike 23
6. Running Shoes, Boots, Sandals, & Insoles 27
   The Anatomy of Footwear 28
   Running Shoes 29
   Hiking Boots 33
   Selecting Hiking Boots 34
   Sandals 37
   Getting a Proper Fit 38
   Customizing Your Footwear 44
   Insoles 45

Part Two: Prevention

7. Making Prevention Work 53
8. The Components of Prevention 55

9. Socks **61**
    Types of Socks 62
    Running Socks 65
    Hiking Socks 68
    Sock Liners 71
    High-Technology Oversocks 72
    Sandal Socks 75
    The Option of Not Wearing Socks 76
10. Powders...**79**
11. Lubricants **81**
12. Skin Tougheners and Tape Adherents **87**
13. Taping for Blisters **91**
    Taping Basics 91
    Duct Tape Techniques 94
    Suzi's Taping Techniques 97
14. 151 Ways to Prevent Blisters **101**
    Things You Do to Your Feet 102
    Things You Apply to Your Feet 103
    Things You Put Around Your Feet......105
    Things You Do in Combinations 108
    Things You Do in General 111
15. Orthotics **115**
16. Nutrition for the Feet **121**
17. Hydration, Dehydration, & Sodium **125**
18. Anti-Perspirants for the Feet.................**129**
19. Gaiters...**133**
20. Lacing Options **139**
21. Changing Your Shoes and Socks **145**
22. Teamwork and Crew Support **149**
    Teamwork 149
    Planning for Footcare.............................150
    Team Responsibilities 151
    Crew Support 151
23. Multi-Day Events **153**

Part Three: Treatments

24. Treatments to Fix Your Feet **159**
25. Hot Spots **161**
26. Blisters **163**
    Blisters 101 164
    Blisters Yesterday, Today, and Tomorrow 166
    General Blister Care 168
    Advanced Blister Care 173
    Extreme Blister Prevention and Care 177
    Beyond Blisters 182
    Fixing Blisters, Their Way or Your Way 183
27. Sprains and Strains, Fractures and Dislocations . **185**
    Sprains and Strains 185
    Ankle Supports 191
    Fractures 194
    Stress Fractures 196
    Dislocations 198
28. Heel Problems **201**
29. Plantar Fasciitis **209**
30. Achilles Tendinitis **217**
31. Stubbed Toes & Toenail Problems **223**
    Stubbed Toes 223
    Toenail Problems 224
32. Morton's Foot & Hammer Toes **229**
    Morton's Foot 229
    Hammer Toes 230
33. Metatarsalgia, Morton's Neuroma,
    & Sesamoiditis **233**
    Metatarsalgia 233
    Morton's Neuroma 235
    Sesamoiditis 237
34. Corns, Calluses, Bunions, & Bursitis **241**
    Corns 241

Calluses 242
Bunions 246
Bursitis 248
35. Numb Toes and Feet 249
   Transient Parasthesia 249
   Peripheral Neuropathy 250
36. Athlete's Foot 253
37. Plantar Warts 255
38. Cold & Heat Therapy 257
39. Foot Care Kits 261

Part Four: Sources & Resources

40. Medical and Footwear Specialists 267
41. Shoe Review and Gear Review Sources 269
42. Internet Feet-Related Web Sites 271
43. Product Sources 273

Glossary 275
Endnotes 279
Bibliography 283
About the Author 285
Index 287

Introduction

This book grew out of my experiences of seeing and hearing the horror stories of athletes who suffer as a result of their foot problems. I have cut the socks off a runner's feet at mile 92 of a 100-mile run and seen the skin fall of the bottoms of both feet. I have helped a runner who completed a 100-mile run and could no longer walk because of the terrible condition of her feet—and literally had to soak the socks off her feet. I have seen the macerated skin on the feet of a runner who failed to take care of his feet through his ultramarathon, and watched the grimacing faces of adventure racers as their teammates tried to repair their horribly blistered and batted feet. I have watched as well-meaning crews and teammates have tried to repair the feet of their fellow athletes and as well-meaning aid station volunteers have tried their best to fix the feet of athletes in their events. In all of these examples, the athletes, crews, and teammates have tried their best—based on their knowledge of what to do, and most often did well. But often there is a better way or other options—and they can be found in the pages of this second edition of *Fixing Your Feet*!

There are few sports that do not use the feet. Most rely heavily on the athlete keeping his or her feet happy and healthy. Many of these athletes have learned the finer points of how to keep their feet in shape. There are many sources of conventional wisdom about footcare and while much of this wisdom is good, the best stuff often comes from athletes who through trial and error, have found unique solutions to what works for their feet—to what is effective in preventing and treating problems. I think Ronald Moak, an Appalachian Trail thru-hiker (1977) and Pacific Crest Trail thru-hiker in 2000, sums it up best, "I would like to think that after 30-years of backpacking, I'd have solved the little dilemma of my feet. But alas I'm not that naive." Ronald has the right idea, it's good to listen to all forms of advice then try different things for yourself. Don't be afraid to go against conventional wisdom. Just because it didn't work for others doesn't mean it won't work for you.

When running, problems with one's feet, whether in a 10K, a duathlon or triathlon, a marathon, or an ultra, are the most common factors that prematurely end or ruin the run. Likewise, in the world of hiking, many a trip has been shortened because of blisters. Adventure racing, typically a unique multi-disciplined sport, requires healthy feet on all team participants at the same time, often over several days. One participant's bad feet can spell disaster for the whole team. Consider the following examples.

Robert Nagel, one of the world's best adventure racers, recalls his experiences in the 1996 Extreme Games, "Our team had a strong and growing lead when my feet caused us to grind to a crawl. We continued, barely, losing over 12-hours in the process, but still managed to take third place." He remembers that ESPN was continuing to show tapes of his feet—16 months after the event! After that experience, he worked hard to perfect a regime that would prevent such a disaster from happening again.

Roland Mueser, in his book *Long-Distance Hiking: Lessons from the Appalachian Trail*, describes what he found when he surveyed hikers. "Problems with feet were endemic. Half of the hikers experienced blisters at the start; many of these were attributed to thrusting tender feet into stiff, heavy boots. During his first few days in Georgia, one hiker was forced into a hospital for an entire week with so many serious blisters that his trip was terminated. And even later when hikers' feet became toughened, the combination of rain, heavy boots, and wet socks meant trouble for one out of five on the trail. One foot-troubled backpacker reported having seven blisters at one time. And more than one hiker, squirming out of boots, was horrified to see socks soaked with blood."[1]

There are no shortcuts to finding what works for each of us. What works for one runner's feet may not work for another runner. The foot care efforts of one hiker or adventure racer may work wonders for him or her but cause you problems. This book offers information that has been tested by experienced athletes: runners, triathletes, adventure runners, hikers, and backpackers. If you study the information and make the application to your specific foot problems, by trial and error, you will determine what works for you. There are hundreds of tips in this book, but the bottom line is that you need to find which ones work for you. Try one. If it doesn't help, try another. Remember though, what works for you today may not work for you tomorrow and what works for me may not work for you.

By doing your homework, you'll be closer to solving your foot problems. If you are constantly plagued by blisters and use a lubricant, try powders; if you use cotton socks, try one of the new synthetic socks or double layer socks; if you use moleskin, try one of the new blister patches. I recommend trying these in your training, not during your competitive events or on your long-awaited hiking trip. Time spent learning what works for your feet can mean more time hiking or running and less time fixing problems when you don't want them or need them.

Two words sum up the advice in this book: *proactive* and *reactive*. Prevention is being *proactive*—working to solve problems before they develop. When problems develop, everything becomes *reactive*—working to solve an existing problem. Being *proactive* takes time up front. Being *reactive* takes time when you often do not have the time or the resources available and may put the event in jeopardy.

Some of you will read the material completely and make intelligent decisions about how to fix your feet. Educating yourself about preventive maintenance and implementing some of the ideas will help reduce your time spent treating problems. Others of you will skip right to the *Treatments* section that describes the problem that you are now having without ever taking the time to read about and understand the components of preventive maintenance. You will very likely continue to have problems until you fully understand the importance of *proactive* prevention before *reactive* treatment.

The real eye-opener, as I researched material and interviewed athletes for the book, even for the second edition, was:

- The extent of the problems so many athletes have with their feet
- That so many of these same athletes naturally expect to have problems
- What has worked for them in the past no longer works
- What they see other athletes do with their feet does not work for them
- They do not know what options they have to fix their feet

This eye-opener led me to: research related books, articles, medical studies; contact numerous companies about their products and services and what they could do for our feet; consult with medical specialists; and talk to runners, hikers, and adventure racers. What I envisioned as a short booklet quickly turned into a book. My office swelled with stacks of product brochures, books, magazines, and boxes of sample products. Encouraged by those I talked to, the project grew.

Dennis Grandy, D.P.M., the Western States 100 Mile Endurance Run Podiatry Director, has treated the foot problems of many hundreds of runners. He has seen "... many conditions that were treated 'on the spot' with no medical reference ever being available. Blisters, although very common, are usually overlooked and often cause the runner to drop from the race." David Hannaford, D.P.M, is a sports podiatrist to many Olympians, ultrarunners, and other endurance athletes. Dr. Bill Trolan has served as medical consultant to adventure racing teams, fixing many participants' feet. Each of these doctors has treated many, many athletes whose runs, hikes, and adventure races are jeopardized because of foot problems. Their experiences underscore the need for this book about *Fixing Your Feet*.

Dave Scott, a good friend and very capable ultrarunner, put the foot problem in proper perspective when he said, "When you don't take care of your feet during a long run or race, each step becomes a reminder of your ignorance." My goal in writing this book is to give you the information necessary to make informed and intelligent choices in both the prevention and treatment of your foot problems.

No matter what your sport, this book can help your with your feet. Whether you are a 10-km runner, a triathlete, a marathoner or an ultrarunner; an overnight hiker or a long-distance thru-hiker; or a novice or veteran multi-sport adventure racer, this book can help you understand how to keep your feet healthy.

Part One

The Basics

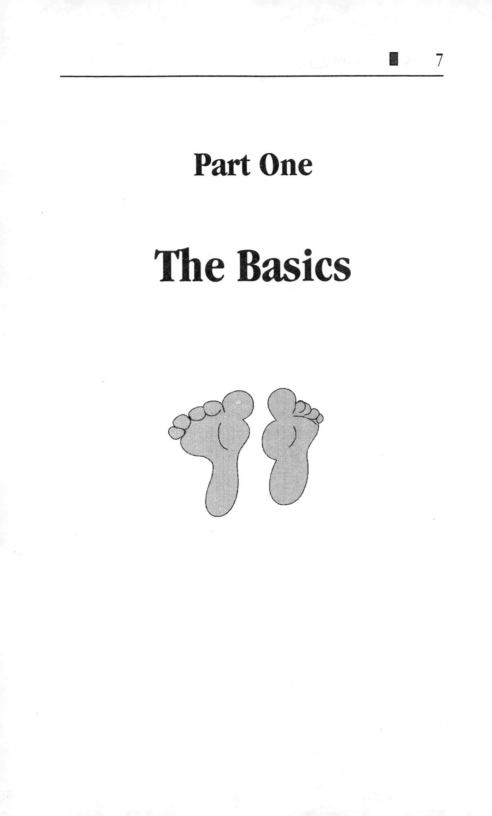

1

Seeking Medical Treatment

The information and advice given in this book is provided to athletes to use in their efforts to resolve foot problems. Not all foot problems or injuries will be resolved successfully by following the tips mentioned in this book.

Never ignore an injury. Pushing through an injury or returning to your sport too early after being injured can lead to additional injuries. You do not want to turn a temporary injury into a permanent disability. Too often athletes rely on self-diagnosis rather than consulting with a medical specialists.

If you have persistent foot problems or recurring pain during or after running or hiking which you cannot resolve, you are advised to seek medical treatment from a medical specialist who can provide his or her medical expertise for your problem. The two main medical specialists for the feet are:

- *Orthopedists* are orthopedic surgeons, experts of the joints, muscles and bones. This includes your upper and lower extremities and the spine. Look for an orthopedist who specializes in the foot and ankle. The American Academy of Orthopaedic Surgeons and the American Orthopaedic Foot and Ankle Society can provide referrals.
- *Podiatrists* are Doctors of Podiatric Medicine (D.P.M.), specialists who work on the feet up to and including the ankles. They specialize in medical and surgical problems including foot diseases, deformities, and injuries. The American

Podiatric Medical Association and the American Academy of Podiatric Sports Medicine can provide referrals.

There is a wide range of skill overlap between orthopedists and podiatrists. Each can treat most of the same foot problems. Talk to them about their training, experience, and whether they have a specialty field. Each of the two specialist area has doctors who specialize in sports medicine. Weigh this information when making a decision about who to turn to for help.

Additionally, there are pedorthists, sports medicine doctors, physical therapists, athletic trainers, massage therapists, and sports chiropractors who can provide assistance for strengthening, alignment, rehabilitation, and footwear design and fit.

- *Pedorthists* work with the design, manufacture, fit, and modification of shoes, boots, and other footwear. Pedorthists who are board certified (C-Ped) to provide prescription footwear and related devices referred by medical specialists. They will evaluate, fit, and modify all types of footwear. The American Orthotics and Prosthetics Association and the Pedorthic Footwear Association can provide information and referrals.
- *Sports medicine doctors* specialize in sports related injuries. They are typically doctors of internal medicine with additional training in sports medicine. When treating athletes with lower extremity injuries that do not improve with their initial treatment, they may refer the athlete to a podiatrist or orthopedist. Most are members of the American College of Sports Medicine (which does not provide referral services).
- *Physical therapists* are licensed to help with restoring function after illness and injury. Most work in close relationship to medical specialists. Physical therapists use a variety of rehabilitation methods to restore function and relieve pain: massage, cold and heat therapy, ultrasound and electrical stimulation, and stretching and strengthening exercises. The American Physical Therapy Association can provide referrals.
- *Athletic trainers* are licensed to work specifically on sports-

related injuries. Rehabilitation methods may be similar to physical therapy but can additionally focus on maintaining cardiovascular fitness while injuries heal. The National Athletic Trainer's Association can provide referrals.

- *Massage therapists* work with athletes in reducing pain and tightness in muscles, tendons, and ligaments—the body's soft tissues. The American Massage Therapy Association can provide referrals.

- *Chiropractors* are doctors of chiropractic medicine who specialize in the alignment of the body's musculoskeletal system. Muscle imbalances, and pelvis, back and neck pain, are often treated by a chiropractor. Some may specialize in sports injuries. Two organizations, the American Chiropractors Association and the International Chiropractic Association can provide referrals.

If you have chronic foot problems, or you are uncertain what your feet are trying to tell you through their pain, consider consulting a podiatrist or orthopedic surgeon. Listen to your whole body and especially your feet. Be attentive to when the pain begins and what makes it hurt more or less. Then be prepared to tell the specialist about the problem, its history, what you have done to correct it, and whether it worked or got worse.

When the time comes to seek medical attention, ask others in your sport for referrals or look in the Yellow Pages. If you have a choice, choose a sports medicine specialist over a general doctor. Information about the associations listed above can be found in the chapter *Medical and Footwear Specialists* on page 267.

2

Sports and and Your Feet

Running, hiking, and adventure racing place extreme demands on our feet. In each of these sports there are wide ranges of difficulty. Where else are our feet forced to put up with such stresses in often ⸴ adverse conditions? Duathlons? Triathlons? Soccer? Court sports? All sports place some degree of extreme stress on our feet.

Running may be a relatively short road 10-km or a grueling ultrarunning event of 100 miles with over 40,000 feet of mountainous ascents and descents. It may be in a short or medium length duathlon or triathlon, or a longer Ironman or Ultraman Triathlon. There are also further extremes: 24-, 48-, and 72-hour runs, six-day runs, and 1000-mile races. The terrain may be paved roads, tracks, fire roads, trails, or cross-country. You may run without any gear, with a single water bottle, or carry a fanny pack loaded with extra socks, food, and waterbottles.

Hiking may be a day trip with a daypack, an overnighter with a mid-weight 40-pound backpack, or a ten-day high-Sierra trip with a pack that tips the scales at 65-pounds. You may be a regular-style backpacker with a full-size pack that carries all the comforts of home. Or you may be a fastpacker with a 30-pound pack or an ultralight backpacker with a 16-pound pack. Regular backpackers may cover six to ten miles in a day, fastpackers may cover 20 miles, while ultralight backpackers can easily cover 30 miles or more. The hike may be an overnighter in your local hills, a week in the desert, a three-week backpack in the Sierras, or a several month thru-hike on the Appalachian Trail or the Pacific Crest Trail.

Adventure racing includes events with names like Eco-Challenge, the Raid Gauloises, or the Beast of the East. These are typically competitive team races with up to five participants who must all finish together. With a combination of sports disciplines like trail or cross-country running, mountain biking, rappelling, climbing, kayaking, canoeing, horse back riding, swimming, glacier climbing, and others, the challenge is an often unknown course with constantly changing terrain. Many are multi-day events over distances up to 300 miles. Paging through several sporting publications I found several of these events advertised. There was the "Hi-Tec Adventure Racing Series," the first nationwide adventure racing series; "The Longest Day Adventure Race," a 32-hour, 100 mile, seven discipline event; the "Eco-Challenge Race Series," a fast-paced, two-day event; and the "Four Winds Adventure Race," a 300-mile, six discipline event. Additionally, individuals experienced in these events are offering training schools to instruct "would-be" adventure racers in the finer points of success across the sport disciplines.

Sport Similarities

What do these sports have in common? The similarities between foot stressing sports are numerous.

- They pound the feet, stress the joints, and strain the muscles, often to unnatural extremes.
- They may take a day, yet often are done over several days, or even a week or more.
- The feet become highly susceptible to hot spots, blisters, and problems with toenails, stubbed toes, bruises, sprains, strains, heel spurs, plantar fasciitis, and Achilles tendinitis.
- The sport can be enjoyed more by solving these common foot problems.

While hikers move slower than runners, the weight of a fully loaded fannypack, lumbar pack, or backpack can easily stress the feet just as the weight a runner places on his or her feet. Adventure racers may stress the feet faster in shorter events and longer over multi-day events because of added stresses from the multi-sport disciplines and the special equipment they may have to carry. The longer multi-day adventure races often tax the feet more than we can imagine with their constant exposure to water or constantly changing adverse conditions.

Studies have shown that "Carrying heavy external loads, (i.e., a heavy backpack) during locomotion appears to increase the likelihood of foot blisters."[2] In addition, the type of physical activity performed is a factor in the probability of blister development. As we intensify our activity and as the duration of the activity increases, frictional forces are increased. Heavy loads, high-intensity activities, and long duration activities describe what we do as runners, hikers, and adventure racers. Most of us perform at least two of these three activities. Ultrarunner Suzie Lister typically experiences few problems with her feet while running ultras. However, when she participated in the 1995 Eco-Challenge the added weight of a pack on her back and the multi-day stresses of adventure racing caused many problems with her feet: blisters-on-top-of-blisters and swollen feet.

The similarities in sports make the preventive maintenance and treatments for blisters and other foot problems work for any sport. The book approaches the different disciplines: running, duathlons and triathlons, hiking and backpacking, and adventure racing, as one-and-the-same when dealing with one's feet. Proper foot care is the most important variable for a successful outing.

3

Conditioning

Conditioning means more than getting your body in condition. It also means getting your feet into the best shape possible for your sport.

Brick Robbins was an adequately trained runner when he started his thru-hike of the Pacific Crest Trail, but quickly found running had not conditioned his feet. The extra weight of a backpack caused additional stress to his feet. By 100 miles his feet were sore and bruised. By the time he reached Idyllwild, another 70 miles, he had "killer" blisters that took another 270 miles to heal. While his feet were in good shape from running, they needed additional conditioning for the weight of a pack.

When Karen Borski thru-hiked the Appalachian Trail in 1998 she had very few foot problems. A year before the thru-hike however, her feet were so out of shape that after an 8-mile day hike they would be riddled with huge blisters on the sides of the heels. Wearing a pack, it only took a few miles before blisters would begin to develop on the soles of her feet, usually the balls of the feet where the main pressure is felt. Karen recalls she was, "So frightened and worried about these blisters that I was afraid I would not be able to thru-hike." To fix the problem she first bought new boots that were slightly too large so that during the course of a hike, as her feet naturally swelled, they wouldn't become too tight and rub. Then she started hiking with a pack every weekend. After hobbling around for most of the following week nursing these awful blisters she would go out and do it again. When calluses finally began to develop, she took up running on the weeknights, both to get her body in shape and to help toughen her feet. Karen found the large calluses on her feet before starting the AT hike helped so she did not have many problems with feet during the trail.

The answer? Your feet must be conditioned to endure the rigors and stresses of whatever sport to which you will be subjecting them. Train in race conditions, in the shoes and socks you will wear on race day. Do short hikes with a pack on your back before taking off to tackle a multi-day hike. Toughen your feet with barefoot walking. Work up to distances that you will tackle in your event. Work out the kinks, find the best shoes and socks for what you will be doing. Learn how to trim your toenails and reduce calluses. Discover the proper insoles that provide support to relieve your plantar fasciitis or heel pain. Strengthen your toes and ankles. In short, do your homework before you head out to tackle the big one. Your feet will thank you.

4

Biomechanics

Biomechanics is the study of the mechanics of a living body, especially of the forces exerted by muscles and gravity on the skeletal
structure. The foot, which includes everything below the ankle, is
a complicated but amazing engineering marvel. With an intricate
biomechanical composition of 26 bones each, together they ac-
count for almost one-quarter the total number of bones in the entire body. There are 33 joints to make the feet flexible. About 20

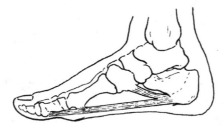

Side view of the bones of foot

Top view of the bones of the foot

muscles manage control of the foot's movements. Tendons stretch
like rubber bands between the bones and muscles so that when a
muscle contracts, the tendon pulls the bone. Each foot contains
more than 100 ligaments that connect bone to bone and cartilage
to bone and hold the whole structure together. Nerve endings make
the feet sensitive. With each step you walk or run, your feet are

subjected to a force of two to three times your body weight, which makes the feet prone to injury.

The big toe, commonly called the *great toe*, helps to maintain balance while the little toes function like a springboard. The three inner metatarsal bones provide rigid support while the two outer metatarsal bones, one on each side of the foot, move to adapt to uneven surfaces.

Your feet are each supported by two arches. The transverse arch runs from side-to-side just back from the ball of the foot. This is the major weight-bearing arch of the foot. The medial longitudinal arch runs the length of the instep, flattening while standing or running and shortening when you sit or lie down, giving spring to the gait. The lateral longitudinal arch runs on the outside of the foot.

Transverse arch

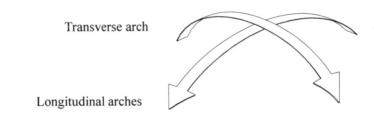

Longitudinal arches

Both longitudinal arches function in absorbing shock loads and balancing the body. These three arches of the foot are referred to singularly as the foot's arch.

Biomechanical Problems

The body lines up over the foot. When the foot goes out of alignment, the ankle, knee, pelvis, and back may all follow. Analyzing the way we stand, walk, and run helps a podiatrist or orthopedist determine whether we have a mechanical misalignment and how it can be corrected. He or she will also want to see your running shoes to analyze the wear patterns on the soles.

An example of biomechanics is how the foot's arch works. A low arch, or flat foot, typically occurs when the foot is excessively pronated, turning it inward. A high arch supinates the foot, rolling it outward. Both of these structural variations can cause knee, hip, and back pain. When one arch flattens more than the other arch, that inner ankle moves closer to the ground. That hip then rotates downward and backward causing a shortening of that leg during walking and running. The pelvis and back both tilt lower on the shortened leg side and the back bends sideways. The opposite leg, which is now longer, is moved outward towards the side that puts added stress on its ankle, knee, and hip. The shoulder on that side then drops towards the dropped hip. All of these are compensations as the body adapts. Muscles, tendons, ligaments and joints are stretched to their limit. The body is out of alignment.

The stresses on our bodies can result in inflammation, often the cause of foot pain. Running on unbalanced and uneven feet may result in fatigue. Fatigue gives way to spasms that may cause a shift in the shape of our feet. Corns, calluses, bunions, spurs, and neuromas may develop when joints are out of alignment.

Do not fall into the trap of drawing erroneous conclusions about your injuries or the type of shoes or equipment that you need for your running style. A podiatrist or orthopedist should check pain associated with running. Heel pain that we try to resolve with a heel pad may not be caused by a heel problem, but by arch problems. This in turn may throw off the biomechanics of the body's alignment. If you begin a run and right away experience knee pain, you most likely have a problem with the knee. If the pain comes after running for a while, it is most likely not a knee problem but a biomechanical problem. Likewise, you may think because you are a heavy runner you need a shoe with lots of cushioning. Based on that decision, you buy a cushioned shoe, the most cushioning insoles, and wear thickly cushioned socks. But, in reality, what you may need is a stability control shoe. This is where the help and expertise of medical specialists comes in. They are trained to determine biomechanical problems.

In 1991, Craig Smith and his brother set out to hike 300 miles of the Continental Divide Trail. With training and planning done, they started with heavy packs that tipped the scale at almost 58 pounds each. Two days and twenty-two miles later Craig had developed severe pain in both knees. Forced to abort the trip, they cached as much gear as possible before starting back. With Craig's knees wrapped with torn T-shirt strips, it took them four days to backtrack the twenty-two miles. It took several weeks of conditioning therapy before he could finally walk without a limp. Craig now packs lighter, does exercises that focus on strengthening the knees, and uses a walking stick on downhills. He could have easily been a victim of biomechanical problems that centered in his knees.

Remember that most athletes have foot problems or become injured by doing too much, too soon, and too fast. To avoid biomechanical problems, use proper footwear, pace yourself, and do strength training.

5

Where You Run and Hike

The terrain is an important part of your running and hiking environment. While a flat, smooth, and resilient surface is ideal, most of us do not have that luxury. Nor do many of us want that type of surface. Most runners spend the majority of their running miles on roads while most hikers spend their time on trails. Variations from our normal running surface can produce problems as we compensate for uphills, downhills, concave surfaces, or irregularities of the surface.

Sidewalks

Concrete sidewalks are harder than any other surface for running. This surface can cause foot, leg or back pain through the jarring of the joints. Care must be taken to watch your footing on sidewalks to avoid the tapered edges of driveways and drop-offs at curbs.

Roads

Road running is the mainstay of most runners. The asphalt surface of most roads provides a softer surface than concrete sidewalks. The problem with roads is the slanted, concave surface curving down towards the sides. Spend a few minutes on your favorite roads to see the angle of their curve and be aware of it. The concave surface puts more stress on the downward side of your shoes and your body. The foot of the higher leg rotates inward while the foot of the lower leg rotates outward. Avoid prolonged running on slanted surfaces. Keep your eyes open for potholes and manhole covers. Of course, the biggest hazard to roadrunners is vehicles. Where possible, run opposite the flow of traffic and safely to one side of the road.

Trails

Trails provide a soft running and hiking surface. Trail running, whether on single-track trails or fire roads, can open new vistas to the adventuresome runner. Whether running or hiking, care must be taken to pay close attention to trail hazards like rocks, roots, wet leaves, mud, etc., all of which can cause a turned ankle or a fall. Trail dust, dirt, pebbles, and rocks can be kicked up into the sock or between the sock and the shoe. These irritants can cause hot spots, blisters, or cuts. Gaiters worn over the shoe or boot tops can help prevent this problem. On rainy days, slippery mud and grasses can present problems with footing. Watch for uneven terrain, roots, and holes on grassy sections of trail.

Hiking on trails while wearing a full backpack presents the added problem of maintaining one's balance with a top-heavy load while negotiating rocks, roots, and uneven trail. Attention to your footing, along with supportive boots, can help prevent a turned ankle. Uphills stretch the Achilles tendons and the calf muscles, and makes the pelvis tilt forward. Downhills increase the impact shock to the heel when landing and tilts the body backward. Continued uphills and downhills may also cause problems with toes, toenails, heel pain, plantar fasciitis, and more.

Tracks

Most runners, at some time, run on tracks. True, they can be boring. Running in circles, actually in ovals, lap after lap after lap after lap may not be your idea of a good run, but there may be a time for it in your running schedule. A track allows us to find out with accuracy how fast we are running. I have used a track for occasional speed workouts. Prior to my first 24-hour track run, I spent three hours running at a local high-school track to "get a feel" for the repetitiveness of track running. The continuous running in one direction stresses the outer leg, so change direction every now and then. Dirt tracks should always be checked for ruts and uneven surfaces that could cause you to trip.

6

Running Shoes, Boots, Sandals, & Insoles

Running and hiking, as far as the feet go, require very little basic equipment. The basics are shoes or boots, socks, and insoles. Yet the war against foot problems can be lost over ill-fitting shoes or boots, socks which cause blisters, or insoles which are not right for your activity. This chapter focuses on running shoes, hiking boots, getting a good fit, and insoles. Sandals are briefly discussed because they are becoming popular. Because socks play such a large role in preventive maintenance, they are discussed at length in the next chapter.

Our feet are unique. Yours may look similar to mine, yet they are as different as our fingerprints. Although our feet may fit into the same size and shape of shoe or boot, there are differences in how our feet actually mold into the shoe. Corns, bunions, susceptibility to blisters, toe length, the type of arches, and the shape of our feet, are just a few of the factors that affect our fit into shoes. Even how we react to and recover from the stresses of running and hiking is important to choosing shoes and boots.

Only you can determine what type of footwear you need to wear. Certainly runners wear running shoes, but there are many types of running shoes. Hikers and adventure racers have many choices in hiking boots but many make the choice to wear running shoes instead of boots. Many of the top teams racing the Eco-Challenge wear running shoes for the whole event, even on snow and ice and while wearing crampons. Just remember the "ifs." If you are used to hiking in running shoes, if your ankles are strong, and if the shoes provide the necessary support while wearing a pack, then running shoes may be right for you. Choose your footwear based on which sport you will be doing, the terrain expected, and your level of experience. Tom McGinnis, who thru-hiked the Appalachian Trail in 1979, makes a good observation, "Good boots and bad socks can be miserable, but cheap boots and good socks can be dreamland." Find the right shoes or boots and the right socks based on what feels right and fits correctly—not by price.

Whether wearing running shoes or boots, remember to inspect them regularly for problems. Frank Sutman was on the second day of a six-day 80-mile backpack trip when one of his boot's outersole split from the midsole to the ball of the foot. He suffered through four days of flapping sole, picking up pebbles, rocks, sticks, and even being tripped up. The moral of his story is to check your boots and shoes before major activities and periodically to keep small problems from becoming major inconveniences. Split outersoles, ripped or torn fabric which lets dirt and rocks into the shoe, cracked heel counters which create folds in the inner heel material, or broken laces retied into a bothersome knot over the top of the foot are all preventable.

The Anatomy of Footwear

By understanding the parts of a shoe or boot, the athlete can make informed choices about which running shoe, crosstrainer, or boot is best for their sport—and for their feet. The parts of a shoe are fairly common, regardless of what kind of shoe you are looking for.

- The shoe's *counter* is the part that wraps around the heel of the foot.
- The *heel* is the back bottom of the shoe.
- The *insole* is the inner insert on which your foot rests. These are typically interchangeable.
- The *outersole* is the shoe's bottom layer.

- The shoe's *shank* is the part of the sole between the heel and the ball of the foot.
- The *toebox* is the tip of the shoe that shapes and protects the toes.
- The *upper* is the top of the shoe that surrounds the foot.

Running Shoes

There are many sources of information about which shoes may be the best for you. The five main sources are the shoe companies, local running stores, running magazines, running catalogs, and running friends. Recognize the difference in the quality of help available from some "chain" shoe stores in shopping malls and that from a store that specializes in running shoes and equipment. A specialized running store usually has personnel who are runners themselves and can watch you run, look at your old shoes, and recommend specific brands of shoes and styles based on what they see and your answers to their questions.

The section *Getting a Proper Fit* on page 38, provides information on how to select a shoe for the best possible fit. To understand running shoes, you need to be aware of their construction. The first construction component is the form over which a shoe or boot is constructed is called a last. Running shoes are built on one of several last patterns.

- *Board* last shoes have the shoe's upper material glued to the shoe's board, which runs the length of the shoe. This generally produces a fairly rigid and stable shoe.
- *Combination* last shoes have the shoe's upper material stitched to either the forefoot (slip-lasted) or the rearfoot (board-lasted). This design offers additional stability at either the footplant or the toe's push-off.
- *Semicurved* lasts are molded straight towards the rearfoot while having some curve towards the forefoot. This mold provides stability and flexibility.
- Semistraight lasts are built to curve slightly from the toe to

the heel. This provides some flexibility and a high degree of stability.

- *Straight* last shoes are built along the shoe's straight arch to provide maximum stability.
- *Slip* last shoes are made with the upper material stitched directly to the midsole without a board. This offers maximum flexibility.

The second construction component is the category that the shoe falls into. There are seven basic categories.

- *Neutral shoes* are made for the runner who has good biomechanics and would be categorized as a neutral pronator. These shoes generally have a good blend of flexibility and stability.
- *Flexibility shoes* are made for runners who are under-pronators, with foot motion towards the outside and who need a shoe which offers more shock-absorbing pronation than their body delivers.
- *Stability shoes* offer high stability and cushioning. Mid-weight or normal arched runners without motion problems who are looking for good cushioning typically use these shoes. These runners usually over-pronate slightly beyond neutral and need a shoe with extra medial support. Most are built on a semicurved last.
- *Motion-control shoes* are those which provide the most control, rigidity, and stability. Heavy runners, severe over-pronators, flat feet runners, and orthotic users often use these shoes. They are typically quite durable shoes but often at a cost of being heavier. Most are built on a straight last and offer the greatest level of medial support.
- *Trail running shoes* are those which usually offer increased toe protection, outsole traction, stability, and durability. Runners who run mainly on trails usually use these shoes.
- *Cushioned shoes* are simply those with the best cushioning. These are typically used by those who do not need extra medial support and by high-arched runners. Most are built on a curved or semicurved last.

- *Lightweight shoes* are those typically made for fast training or racing. These come with varying degrees of stability and cushioning and can be worn by runners with little or no foot problems. Most are built on a curved or semicurved last.

Once you buy a new pair of shoes, wear them around the house to be sure they fit well and are comfortable. Herb Hedgecock bought a pair of New Balance 827s and found the uppers rubbed against his ankles, making them sore. Later models seem to have resolved the problem. If you sense problems, return the shoes for another style or type. Even the same shoe model that you have worn in the past can have a minor design changes in a new release. Wear them for a while until you are sure they fit well.

Sometimes shopping for running shoes can be mind boggling. In a Dilbert cartoon in the Sunday Comics, we were reminded of the humor in buying shoes.

- Frame 1. Dilbert is looking over shoes on a sale rack.
- Frame 2. The salesman asks, "Do you have any questions?"
- Frame 3. Dilbert responds, "What's your best running shoe?"
- Frame 4. The salesman says, "They're all the same. Sneakers are sneakers."
- Frame 5. The boss says to the salesman, "Alan, may I have a word with you?"
- Frame 6. They talk behind Dilbert's back as he looks at shoes.
- Frame 7. The salesman now says, "The expensive sneakers are far superior." Dilbert responds, "I'll take them."
- Frame 8. The salesman thinks to himself, "I feel like I'm clubbing a baby seal." as Dilbert asks "Will these work with my old socks?"

Shoe designs are always changing. Often our favorite shoes disappear from the shelves and we find ourselves forced to make new choices. Do your homework, study the shoe reviews and the ads, talk to your running friends, and try them on. Good stores will let you run in them. Orin Dahl once found that his favorite shoes were no longer offered. Instead of the old shoes, Nike offered a new type of "air" shoe. He bought the shoes and began running in them. The new shoes were not as flexible in the forefoot causing his heel to pull up and out of the shoe. To his dismay, he developed blisters at the back of his heels. He recalls how he turned the shoes over to the Salvation Army and began a search for a different pair. He has no doubt that the shoes were good shoes. They were just not right for his feet and running style. As you look for shoes, remember that not every pair of shoes is right for your feet. Consider the following experience of Jeff Washburn.

I did ten 100's in 1999. Rocky Raccoon, Umstead, Massanutten, Old Dominion, Western States, Vermont, Leadville, Wasatch, Angeles Crest and Arkansas.

I really didn't have too much of a problem with my feet last year. The Rocky Racoon (the first one) is where I had the most trouble. It was 80 degrees and very humid and I wore my last year's shoes which were size eleven (my normal size). Since the shoes were a bit worn and because of some swelling because of the humidity, I had several blisters between my toes. After the run, I drained them with a pin and then pretty much forgot about them. They dried and peeled within a week or two.

I then bought some Asics 2040's and Montrail Vitesse shoes in a size twelve. I always wear double-layer, blister-free socks. The rest of the way, I had very little blister problems. The only consistent blister problem was with the Montrails. If I didn't put duct tape on the balls of my feet, they would develop blisters. They also rubbed on the outside of my left big toe. I did not need any tape with the 2040's. Even at the hot and humid Vermont 100, I had little problem with blisters (mostly as a result of wearing the Montrails). On rare occasions, I would get a small blister on the inside of the big toe on my right foot.

I never put anything on my feet. I do, however, use Succeed electrolyte caps. This has helped me with stomach distress (I only drink water or, late in the race, Pepsi). I am sure that it also helps with the blistering but I can't confirm whether it is the larger shoe size or the caps since I did use the caps at Rocky Raccoon. I also had a fever at Rocky Raccoon which may have contributed some to my blistering there. I think experience has a lot to do with blisters. The more races I run the tougher my feet become. I think swelling (caused by the constant pounding) also contributes.

Hiking Boots

My first pair of hiking boots were all leather, with thick Virbram soles, laced all the way to my calf, and seemed to weigh as much as my loaded backpack. Times have changed and so have hiking boots. Because of technology, they fit better and are easier on your feet. Running shoe technology has had a positive influence on hiking boots. Insoles, molding, padding, and midsole and outersole advances have made many of them as comfortable as lighter-weight boots. A recent ad by bootmaker Sorel claimed, "Any boot can repel water. Ours will actually suck the sweat off your pinky toes." As technology advances, many bootmakers, like Sorel, will offer moisture control systems to wick perspiration away from your feet. Gor-Tex fabrics are commonly built into boots for moisture transfer. Lacing systems are also changing for the better.

Many hikers have been converted to using the newer light-weight boots. These are usually as flexible as running shoes and carry many of the running shoe benefits of fit and comfort. Because of their flexibility and construction, many of these require very little or no break-in time. I completed an 8.5-day, 221-mile ultra-light backpack of the John Muir Trail in regular running shoes. Unless you are used to hiking or running trails in running shoes while wearing a backpack, I do not recommend them for backpacking. Since I did the John Muir Trail in 1987, boots have changed. Today, I would consider a trail running shoe or light-weight boot for the same hike.

Check out some of the features of new hiking boots at your local store. Many boots offer a combination of features: lighter weight, breathable uppers, high-traction and long-lasting outersoles, improved lacing systems, flexible footbeds, stable and cushioning midsoles, wider toe boxes, and Gore-Tex fabric incorporated into the uppers. Boots can be rated in three categories: lightweight hiking—for trail hiking and light loads; midweight hiking—for on/off trail hiking and light backpacking; and heavyweight hiking—for on/off trail, heavy loads, and multi-day trips. First, determine the type of hiking you will be doing and how much support and protection you will need for the weight you will carry. Second, look at the various features of different boots in each of the three categories. Then shop accordingly, but do not rule out a certain type of boot until you try them on your feet. A boot that pinches or rubs in the store will not feel better when you are out on the trail. Rob Langsdorf suggests taking time to really test a new boot before leaving the store. He shares, "I usually wear mine around the store for an hour or more before deciding to take it. It takes time, but consumes less time than having to return it or having to spend lots of time treating blisters. Then break new boots in by wearing them around the house, to work, church, etc. before going out on the trail. Begin with easy hikes before starting off on a long trip. Only when they feel good on a short hike are they ready for a longer one."

Many boots still need to be broken in. Rob adds, "I had a friend who bought a pair of boots, but didn't break them in because she felt that wearing them around the house wasn't the feminine thing to do. She ended up with major blisters after 6-7 miles. Buy the end of our 15-mile weekend backpack she was ready to throw the new boots away and swear off ever backpacking again. All because she didn't want to look funny wearing her boots in town."

Once you have your boots, be sure they still fit after not wearing them for a while. Take at least one break in walk in them before going on a major hike. Your feet may have changed and they may need to get reacquainted with the boots before a long hike.

Selecting Hiking Boots

Before buying boots, check *Backpacker* and *Outside* magazines for their coverage on hiking boots. These articles evaluate most brands based on fixed standards while identifying their features and costs. Then check out your local backpacking supply store for the brands and styles they carry. Spend as much time as is necessary to get a good fit. Tell the salesperson what type of hiking you will be doing, for how long, and how much weight you plan on carrying. Try on several pairs of boots by different companies. Use your own socks. Walk in the boots. Squat in them. Look for a pair that fits right from the start and grips your heels. Take out the insoles and look at the boot's construction. Find the pair that fits and feels better than the others. Purchase a high-quality boot made for hiking rather than lightweight boots sold for general-purpose street wear. These "fashion-statement" boots will not hold up under the stresses of heavy trail use. Utilize the experience of the personnel of your local camping and backpacking stores to help you in making a wise decision, but realize the final decision is yours based on how they feel on your feet.

Remember that the boots you select will each be picked up and put down many times each day. Hiking 12 miles each day would equate to 25,000 steps[3], day after day. Feel the weight of your boot and think about each step. Heavier boots are not always the best. True, they may provide more ankle stabilization, but you could get more benefit from a lightweight boot and proper ankle and foot strength conditioning before the hike. Ray Jardine, who has hiked the Pacific Crest Trail three times and the Appalachian and Continental Divide Trails each once, estimates that each 3.5 ounces off a pair of boots will add about a mile to a day's hiking progress.[4] A review of one store's boot selection showed weights for a pair of boots ranging from one pound nine ounces all the way to three pounds nine ounces. Selecting boots that weigh 10.5 ounces less than another pair could mean an additional three miles hiked per day. An educated choice based on boot features, your personal needs, and the terrain ahead is necessary.

Ed Acheson made several painful discoveries when he hiked the Pacific Crest Trail. With his boots not completely broken in, he switched to a different pair on a salesperson's recommendation. The boots were too much boot for him and a half size too small—the salesperson told him they were sized larger than most. Ed remembers for the first 20 days having "... more blisters than the number of days I had been out." Because of the blisters he compensated his gait which in turn gave him knee problems. Before he could get new boots he was forced to cross the Mojave in tennis shoes. He still suffers from problems he attributes to the wrong boots.

Some boot companies, like Merrill and Vasque, have developed what they call their "Hiking Boot Last" which is designed to be snug around the heel and arch, and with a roomy toe box. Both offer three different insoles for a better fit, and the use of different thicknesses of socks and the number of pair's worn to adjust the fit even more.

If you are planning a several-week hike or a several-month thru-hike on a multi-state trail, remember the need to buy boots larger than normal to accommodate your feet as they become stronger and enlarge to their normal hiking size. Try on boots that are anywhere from one to two sizes larger than normal, which will allow your feet to fit into them properly.

Some boots will soften and become more flexible with forceful flexion of the soles and uppers, hand-working of waterproofing solution into the leather, or mechanical flexion of the uppers at a shoe shop. If your boots are too stiff try one of these three methods.

A week into hiking the John Muir Trail, Andrew Ferguson developed a "hellatious" deep blister on the back of his right foot, about 1.5″ in diameter. By nursing the blister with Spenco 2nd Skin and tape he hiked for three days in running shoes before reaching civilization and purchasing a new pair of boots. The red heel bothered him for two weeks and took six months to return to normal. Andrew is now a believer in running shoes for hiking. Many people prefer running shoes instead of boots for hiking.

If you are always having problems with your boots and a different set of boots does not help, consider trying a pair of running shoes, preferably trail running shoes. Be aware, however, of the differences. Running shoes do not provide the same degree of ankle support and overall foot protection. While some may prefer the increased ankle mobility in a low running shoe, this choice requires proper strength in the feet, ankles, and legs. My choice to wear running shoes when fastpacking the 221 miles of the John Muir Trail was based on a trial overnight hike with a full backpack and years of running trails. I knew my feet and ankles could handle the stresses of the trail in running shoes and I did not need heavier boots.

When you do have problems with your feet, and you usually

will at some point, you need to look at the boots and evaluate whether you need to replace them with another boot type and/or style. On long hikes, your feet do enlarge and change. Boots wear out. Over a couple of years your feet may also change. Be open to new styles and features in newer type boots and find the pair that best fits you.

Sandals

Tired of running shoes that fit him poorly, caused blisters and toe-nail problems, and seemed to collect dirt, Rob Grant bought a pair of sandals. He used his Teva Terradactyls in a Sri Chinmoy 24-Hour Run. At 100 km both small toes were swollen. The next day he ground down the ridge on the footbeds that fits under the toes. This corrected the problem. After putting 405 miles on the sandals, he reports no noticeable wear on the soles or the straps. Rob found that rubbing Vaseline on the inside of the straps helped to soften then when first used. He feels that ankle support in sandals is comparable to that of running shoes.

Sandals are becoming more popular as designs improve to provide better traction, foot control, and comfort. Changing from running shoes or hiking boots into an open pair of sandals can be refreshing. When your feet are tired, hot, or sore, sandals can feel like a small piece of heaven on earth.

Hikers and backpackers can benefit from sandals. Jerry Goller backpacked in Merrell or Teva sandals for five years. He reports, "I use them in winter (with Seal Skins and fleece socks) and summer. My feet are actually warmer than when I hiked in boots. They are much more comfortable and, of course, lighter. Stream fording is easier. Ankle support is overrated—sandals work just fine for my feet." Jerry's longest backpack wearing sandals is 800 miles!

When shopping for sandals, try several designs. The straps may rub you wrong. A different style may offer straps that fit better. Some strapping systems require readjustment each time you put them on. If you will be wearing socks with them, be sure they have adequate space for your socks. Look at the soles for adequate traction design. Some designs offer a lip around the edge of the sandal that can provide a degree of protection from rocks and roots.

Teva has a new sandal, the Teva Wraptor, advertised as the "... world's first performance running sandal." Using a patent-pending strapping system and a Fusion Arch, the sandal offers "... unparalleled adjustability, comfort, and control." The strapping system flexes to adjust to the runner's arch and assist in motion control. Those who prefer the freedom of sandals over constricting shoes may find the Wraptor to their liking.

Wearing sandals while running or hiking takes getting used to. Small pebbles, gravel, leaves, or other debris can easily work their way underfoot. Shaking the foot or a light kick against a rock will usually knock these loose. Be especially careful of sticks on the trail that could inflict a puncture wound to your exposed feet. If you wear sandals without socks the skin of the foot will eventually toughen into calluses. Check the calluses regularly for cracks that can split through to uncallused skin and bleed or become infected.

Products

Wraptor Sandal   The Wraptor is a unique sandal made for running. With a raised toe spring to protect from rocks, roots, and debris; a dual density EVA midsole with a molded shank arch plate; a Heel Shoc Pad; a quick dry upper; and a heavily lugged Traction Rubber bottomsole, this sandal will work well on trails and roads. With a contour molded, waterproof sueded footbed, the sandal should be comfortable in bare foot. Teva Sport Sandals, PO Box 968, Flagstaff, AZ 86002; (800) 376-8382; www.teva.com.

Getting a Proper Fit

Karen Berger, in *Advanced Backpacking*, makes a good comment on the fit of boots—and the same advice applies to running shoes. "Like most marriages, the mesh between boot and foot is not always a good match. If you look at the feet of several people, you'll undoubtedly see a range of bumps and bunions, arches and ankle-bones—all of which are encased in the same hard leather cage. It takes a bit of time, accommodation, and softening for boots and feet to settle into comfortable routine."[5] There are many factors to a good fit.

Rich Schick, a Physician's Assistant and ultrarunner, believes the key to getting the proper size shoe is the insert, "If the foot does not fit the insert, then the shoe will have to stretch to accommodate the difference or there may be excessive room in the shoe, which can lead to blisters and other foot problems." He thinks there is too much confusion about straight lasts, curved lasts, semi-curved lasts etc., "You don't need to know any of this if you use the insert to fit your shoes. The same holds true for the proper width of shoe. Simply remove the insert from the shoe and place your heel in the depression made for the heel. There should be an inch to an inch and a half from the tip of you longest toe to the tip of the insert. None of your toes or any part of the foot should lap over the sides of the insert. If they do, is it because the insert is too narrow or is it because of a curved foot and straight insert or vice versa? The foot should not be more than about a quarter inch from the edges of the insert either. This includes the area around the heel or the shoe may be too loose. Check to see if the arch of the insert fits in the arch of your foot. Finally, if all the above criteria are met then try on the shoe. About the only remaining pitfalls are a tight toe box and seams or uppers that rub."

Many shoe and boot companies suggest which of their models are best for certain types of activities, certain types of feet, and certain types of runners or hikers. They do that because many shoes are made for a specific type of foot—and many people have feet which will work with one type of shoe better than another type. Look for the *Runner's World* shoe-buyer's guides, the *Trail Runner* and *Running Times* shoe reviews, *Backpacking* magazine's boot reviews, and *Outside* magazine's Buyer's Guide for helpful information.[6] Other sport-specific magazines may offer similar reviews. With knowledge of biomechanics and your specific foot type, you can make a better choice than shopping blindly. When shopping for shoes or boots, try on several different pairs, by several different companies. This will help you identify those that feel good initially versus those that just don't feel quite right. Knowing how different shoes and boots fit your feet will help in the final selection.

A biomechanically efficient runner lands on the back outside of the heel and rolls inward (pronation) to absorb shock, with the foot flattening as the motion moves forward, rolls through the ball of the foot and rotates outward (supination) to the push off. Over-pronation is the inward roll of the foot as you roll off the heel. Supination is the outward roll of the foot as you push off the toe.

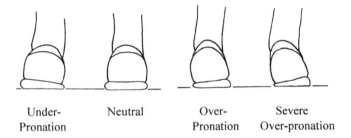

| Under-
Pronation | Neutral | Over-
Pronation | Severe
Over-pronation |

Depending on whose advice you take when looking for shoes, you may do one of several things.

- Have a friend watch you walk or run or even videotape your feet to determine how they land, how much you pronate, and your general form. This, with the wear patterns on your old shoes, can help determine whether you should look for shoes which compensate for under-pronation, over-pronation, severe over-pronation, or whether can get by with shoes for neutral pronators. Use this information to select shoes from one of four categories: flexibility trainers for under-pronators, neutral trainers for neutral pronators, stability trainers for over-pronators, and motion-control trainers for severe over-pronators.[7]
- First match your running and biomechanical needs, including your most common running surface into one of five categories: motion-control, stability, cushioned, lightweight training, or trails. Secondly, determine whether your foot type is normal, flat, or high-arched (found below). Use this information to select shoes from that category.[8]

Take your old shoes with you when you shop for new shoes. The wear patterns on the soles can help you, or the salesperson, determine how you run and the best shoes for your running style. Normal wear is on the outer heel and the across the ball of the foot. Pronators show wear on the outer heel and the inner forward side of the shoe. Supinators typically show wear on the heel to the forefoot along the outer edge of the shoe.

The key to getting a good fit in running shoes is to know your foot type. To determine your foot type, walk on a hard surface with wet, bare feet to see your imprint. You should fit one of three arch types.

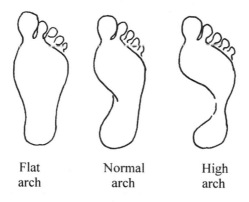

Flat   Normal   High
arch   arch   arch

- *Normal arched feet* leave an imprint that shows the forefoot and heel connected, but with an inward curve at the arch. These runners will typically do best in a semicurved last shoe since they are generally efficient in their running gait and do not need motion-control shoes.
- *Flat-arched feet* leave an imprint that is almost complete without an inward curve at the arch. These runners will typically do best in a semicurved or straight last shoe that offers good stability and/or motion control. These runners are often overpronators.
- *High-arched feet* leave an imprint that shows the forefoot and heel connected by a very narrow curve at the arch. These runners will typically do best in a curved last shoe with good cushioning. These runners are often supinators (under-pronators).

Shop around until you find running shoes that feel right on your feet. A correct fit will help in blister prevention. Valerie Doyle remembers her fight to beat blisters. When she learned how to buy shoes that fit properly she found they solved her blister problem. The same applies to fitting boots. Studies have found that tight footwear can increase the forces exerted by the shoe or boot on the foot, increasing blister probability, while loose-fitting footwear increases the movement of the foot inside the shoe or boot, causing increased friction forces on the foot, which in turn increases blister probability.[9] Walk in the boots for a while to be sure they are comfortable and do not have any pressure points. Some shoes and boots will be higher at the ankle and may put pressure on your foot. Others will not bend at the same forefoot and toe point, making an uncomfortable heel to toe transition or pinching the toes. There may also be a seam inside the shoe or boot that rubs your foot and creates pressure and a potential blister. Pay close attention to the overall fit.

You may find shoes that fit well with one exception. The toes may pinch or you may have corns or bunions that create pressure in specific areas. Some runners will cut slits into the side or the toe boxes of shoes to provide a better fit. Other runners will actually cut out a portion of the shoe over the problem area. If you do this, be careful not to sacrifice the integrity of the shoe. Be aware of the additional problem this may cause. Dirt and small rocks can easily get into the shoe and lead to hot spots and blisters.

If you have narrow or wide feet, consider shopping for shoes or boots that offer variable lacing capabilities. These shoes and boots will have lace eyelets that are not lined up in an up-and-down row but spaced horizontally farther apart. See the chapter *Lacing Options* on page 139 for information on how to lace for different types of feet.

The American Academy of Orthopaedic Surgeons gives suggestions for buying shoes. Foremost, they remind us that shoes should always conform to the shape of your feet, your feet should never be forced to conform to the shape of a pair of shoes. Their suggestions apply equally well to buying boots. Suggestions include:

- Fit new shoes to your larger foot. Have your feet sized each time you buy new footwear.
- Try on and fully lace both shoes.
- Judge a shoe by how it fits on your foot, not by the marked size.
- Try on shoes at the end of the day, preferably after running or walking, because your feet normally swell and become larger after standing and sitting during the day.
- Wear the same type of socks that you will wear for running or hiking.
- You should be able freely to wiggle all your toes.
- There should be a firm grip of the shoe to your heel.
- Make sure you do not feel the seams or stitching inside the shoes.

When you purchase footwear, consider the whole picture, not just the shoe or boot you hold in your hand. Hiker Pat Radney has learned, the hard way, that your footwear must work with your choice of socks, insoles, orthotics (if your wear them), and with the activity you will be using them for. Walking around the store in a pair of hiking boots that feel OK may change when you get home and try them when carrying a 30-40 pound pack on your back.

Long-distance hikers may find their feet enlarging by one or more sizes while on a long thru-hike. Ultrarunners typically find themselves needing larger shoes, often by several sizes, during a multi-day event. Remember to allow enough toe space when buying either shoes or boots. Allow about a 1/2" space between the end of the longest toe and the front of the shoe. When the foot is in the shoe, the arch naturally flattens. Since the heel is held in place by the heel of the shoe, the foot can only move forward. If the shoe does not have this bit of extra space in the toe box, the toes become cramped. Toenail problems, blisters, and calluses may develop. This important consideration is the fit problem most often overlooked.

Customizing Your Footwear

When you shop for shoes or boots, run your fingers around the inside to determine whether there are any rough spots, overlapping or raised seams, or other potential pressure points that could cause hot spots or blisters. These may be able to be rubbed flat or softened. Ask the store for another pair to determine if the spots are common to that style or just one particular shoe or boot. If these spots are common to that particular shoe or boot, you may have to customize your footwear for a good fit.

Buck Jones has found this means if a shoe or boot has any ledges, ridges, or extrusions around the ankle or heel, they will rub into your feet and potentially cause a problem. These extrusions my be their due to stitches, extra foam, or by design. The contour around your heel and ankle has to be smooth from the base of your foot all the way up to your ankle or the top of your heel. Buck has had two such experiences. In the first, while an hour into a short hike in his new pair of trail running shoes he discovered the shoes had made a hole in his sock and was working on his ankle. He recalls, "I applied duck tape and moleskin to my foot and also patched the shoe with duck tape and moleskin so that the ledge was minimal." He was able to finish his hike with little more wear on his foot. His second experience was with a friend. She was a beginner hiker and shortly after starting a hike was bothered by a hot spot. It was similar to what Buck had experienced. The boot had a stitch around the heel and it was causing a blister. Buck applied duck tape and moleskin on the foot and under the void of the stitch. By mending both the foot and the shoe they were able save the foot from further damage. Now before he buy a pair of shoes, the first thing he looks for is a bad design around the heel and ankle area.

If you have difficulty finding quality shoes that fit your particular type of foot problems, consider searching for a certified pedorthist. A pedorthist is an individual trained to work on the fit or modification of shoes and orthotics to alleviate foot problems caused by disease, overuse, or injury. He or she may be able to modify your running shoe(s) or boot(s), internally or externally, for a better fit. Look in the telephone book or ask your orthopedist or podiatrist for references. The chapter *Medical and Footwear Specialists* on page 267 has information on the Pedorthic Footwear Association.

Insoles

Insoles are designed to provide extra support and/or cushioning during running and hiking. Some models are molded to cradle the heel, support the arch, and cushion the forefoot while others have only an arch support, or are flat. Replacement insoles are to be used in place of your shoe's standard insole. Many replacement insoles offer better heel support, shock absorption, energy return, and reduction of friction than the insoles that come with the shoes. Some have a better arch support that will help with flat feet problems. The insoles listed below are typically found in running, camping, and sporting goods stores. Ask to see their product catalogs if their shelf stock is low or if you are looking for a particular type. Some stores offer custom made insoles which may provide a better fit than a general insole.

There are basically two types of insoles available, foam and viscous polymer. The foam has the advantages of lightweight less, heat retention and inexpensive. Its disadvantages are that it is not near as good of an impact absorber, and it loses its impact absorbing properties with use. In general foam is more suited for runners because of the concern about weight. The viscous polymers are a great choice for hikers, especially in rocky terrain. Rich recommends the polymer insoles for runners with sensitive feet or injuries where the padding would protect the area. There are hybrid inserts available that offer polymer at the heel and/or forefoot and the remainder of the insert in foam. This reduces the weight liability.

If you have tried changing socks and other techniques to decrease your chance of blisters, try changing insoles. You may find that a particular brand or type of insole may be better at reducing blisters on your feet. This is usually due to the fabric or components of the insole. Insoles are not made to last forever. Check them for breakdown and replace them when necessary. This will depend on how you run and hike, and your mileage. Replacement insoles may be sized differently. Be sure to check the fit inside your shoes or boots for a good fit. An insole that is narrow in the forefoot can create problems as the foot overlaps space between the narrow insole and the side of the shoe. Insoles may be different in other areas also. Some may have a higher arch that will put pressure on your foot, creating blisters. Others may have a narrow heel bed and cause friction where your foot rubs against the top edge of the heel cup. Finding and using the right insole can make a big difference in the overall fit and comfort of your footwear.

Replacement insoles are not sold as corrective footbeds. If a particular brand or style of insole is uncomfortable or causes pain, try another type. One brand may fit your feet better than another brand. Some are quite rigid while others are very cushioned. Try several until you find a pair that is comfortable for your activity. Do not confuse these insoles with an orthotic. Always consult with a pedorthist, orthopedist, or podiatrist if you are having frequent foot problems.

If you purchase insoles and they are too tight in certain areas of your feet, inquire with your local shoe repair shop or a pedorthist about thinning them with a belt sander.

If your feet tend to slip around inside your shoes, TacLiner insoles and TacTape may help control slippage. These unique products are made with a motion control slip resistant lining/tape that "... gently holds the foot in the proper position in the shoe, preventing blisters and turf toe as well as reducing pronation."

Repeated foot pain may be a sign of deeper foot problems that a general use insole cannot correct. See the chapter *Orthotics* on page 115 for information on custom-made and over-the-counter orthotics.

Products

The insoles listed below are a sampling of what is available to the general public. New models and designs are constantly being introduced. Check your local running, hiking, and footwear stores for a current offering.

Arch Crafters Custom-Fit Insoles   These insoles are an example of what some stores offer to the general public. They are often used as a substitute for orthotics. AmFit uses a scanned image of your feet to make a custom insole. To find a store near you that uses this technology, contact AmFit Inc., 2850 Bowers Avenue, Santa Clara, CA 95951; (408) 986-1232; www.amfit.com.

DRYZ Insoles   These insoles help the feet stay dryer and cooler while eliminating odor. The wicking sock liner transports the foot's perspiration and moisture into an inner layer of copolymer foam that absorbs and stores the moisture in a gel-like substance. The gelled moisture dissipates continuously throughout the day and completely when your shoes are removed. Their sport insoles are engineered for enhanced comfort, cushion, and performance. For more information contact Dicon Technologies, 3-00 Banta Place, Fairlawn, NJ 07410; (877) 342-6685; www.dryz.com.

Hapad Comf-Orthotic   Hapad makes full-length and 3/4-length insoles. The original contoured Comf-Orthotic full-length and 3/4-length insoles are made from Hapad featherweight wool. The coiled, spring-like wool fibers provide firm and resilient support while providing arch, metatarsal, and heel cushioning. The full-length contoured Comf-Orthotic Sports Replacement Insole is made in three layers with a moisture wicking suede top, a ventilated Poron middle layer for shock absorption, and a bottom of Microcel "Puff," a self-molding footbed. The insole includes a metatarsal bar to relieve pressure at the ball of the foot, a medial arch support to limit pronation, and a heel cup for stability and control of the foot and ankle. For more information contact Hapad, Inc., PO Box 6, 5301 Enterprise Blvd., Bethel Park, PA 15102; (800) 544-2723; www.hapad.com.

Second Wind   Second Wind makes several different types of insoles with good cushioning. The Air^2 and Flat Foot Insoles, and others. For more information contact Second Wind Products, PO Box 2300, Paso Robles, CA 93447; (800) 248-0425; www.2ndwind.com.

Sof Sole   Sof Sole by IMPLUS is a line of replacement insoles made with the Implus Cellular Cushioning System. This open-cell material provides superior shock absorption while allowing air and moisture to pass through. Additionally, these insoles contain a biocide additive to retard the growth of bacteria and fungus. Choose from Sof Motion Control, Sof Athletes Plus, and others. For more information contact IMPLUS Corporation, 4900 Prospectus Drive, Suite 300, Durham, NC 27713; www.sofsole.com.

Spenco   Spenco makes several types of replacement insoles for runners. Choose from a molded full length cushioning system of Polysorb for best shock absorption and energy return, in several styles: Walker/Runner, Hiker/Casual, Court/Aerobic, etc. Also offered is a closed cell neoprene arch cushion in full- or 3/4-length, a Slip-In flat insole, and a full-length Gel Cushion Insole. For sports involving rapid stopping and starting, Spenco offers the Turfsole Sport Insoles with stiff spring steel insert combined with Maxxon urethane. For more information contact Spenco Medical Corporation, PO Box 2501, Waco, TX 76702-2501; (800) 877-3626; www.spenco.com.

Spectrum Sports   Spectrum Sports makes an assortment of replacement insoles. Choose from the Ultra Sole, Graphite Arch, Ultra Sole, Sorbo Lite and Sorboair made with Sorbothane, all made with a visco elastic polymer with high impact shock absorption. Other insoles include the Silver Liner made from a lightweight polyurethane foam, the Summit Hiking and Backpacking insole with Sorbothane, or a neoprene 3/4-length arch support. For more information contact Spectrum Sports, Twinsburg, OH 44087; www.sorbothane-spectrum.com.

Superfeet   Superfeet footbeds are made in three systems: trim-to-fit, replacement-fit, and custom-fit. Their corrective shape and design offers a stabilizer cap which provides excellent support and stability to the bone structure of the foot, allowing the foot muscles to function more efficiently. In the trim-to-fit system, the low and high profile models are made for running and hiking. Replacement system footbeds are the lower end of the line without the stabilizer cap. For information on stores that have the custom-fit system, contact Superfeet Worldwide, 1419 Whitehorn St., Ferndale, WA 98248; (800) 634-6618; www.superfeet.com.

TacLiner Insoles   These insoles are made with a slip resistant surface from triple density foam for maximum shock absorption, are moisture absorbing, and breathable. They hold the foot in position inside the shoe or boot. Unaffected by water, the tape will hold its slip resistant features under any weather conditions. For more information contact TacLiner Footwear & Athletic Products, 14460 Cadillac Drive, San Antonio, TX 78248; (210) 479-5588; www.tacliner.com.

TacTape   This unique tape comes on a roll that is 10 yards long by 1 3/4 inches wide. TacTape stretches in its width, but not in its length, helping to maintain the foots position in the shoe. The tape can be applied to any insole, orthotic, or the bottom of your shoe, boot, or sandal. It can also be used on the shoe's tongue or as a foot wrap directly on the skin or over the sock. Unaffected by water, the tape will hold its slip resistant features under any weather conditions. For more information contact TacLiner Footwear & Athletic Products as listed above.

Other Insole Sources   Some boot companies like Merrell and Vasque also make insoles. Check your local store for these and other insoles. Many drug stores and pharmacies also stock insoles.

Part Two

Prevention

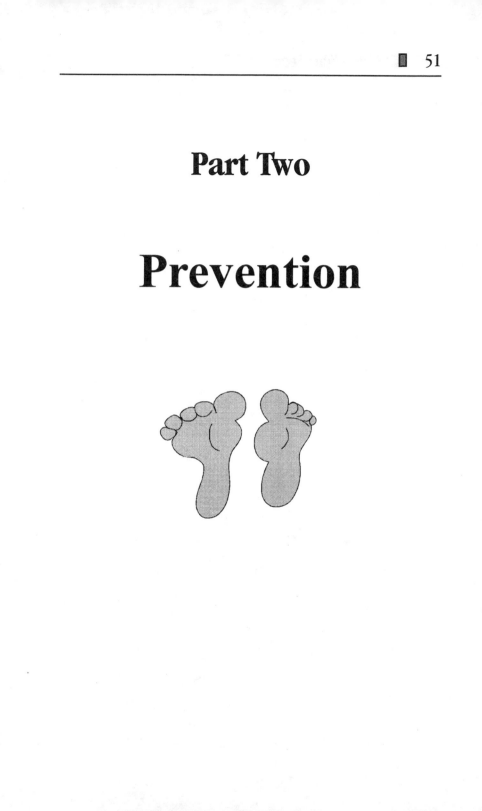

7

Making Prevention Work

"The 6th Law Of Running Injuries:
Treat the Cause, Not the Effect.
Because each running injury has a cause, it follows
that the injury can never be cured until the causative
factors are eliminated."
Tim Noakes, MD, *The Lore of Running*.[10]

Tim Noakes' 6th Law of Running Injuries must be remembered—
any running injury can be cured *only* after the cause is found and
eliminated. All of us who run, hike, or adventure race at some
point have problems or injuries with our feet. This section on prevention is lengthy because there are many factors that can help
prevent the cause of foot problems and injuries. Prevention is the
key to saving one's feet.

Prevention is *proactive*. Time spent being proactive in preventing problems will pay off in the long run. Taking a *proactive*
approach will mean less time being *reactive* to problems when
you often do not have the time to spare nor readily available materials.

The key to making prevention work is to find what works for
you in the environment where you will use it. In other words, try
the fix where it will be used. When you are trying to find what
works for you on trails, running on roads will not typically provide the same results as actually running on trails. I made my own
gaiters for trail running after determining that the dirt getting into

my shoes was causing hot spots and blisters. I never would have made that determination without running on trails. Likewise, walking around town while wearing a backpack and your hiking boots is never the same as hiking on a rocky trail with uneven terrain. That may help to break in the boots but will not give the same feeling as a rough rocky trail.

Your feet will respond to training in the same way your legs respond. Increasing your running or hiking time by increments will allow your feet time to adapt to the added stresses of the additional mileage. Suddenly doubling your mileage will likely lead to potential problems. If you are working up to a marathon, an ultra, longer ultras, or a multi-day hike, do back-to-back training days to work your feet into their best possible condition.

Mike Palmer has spent years finding what works for his feet. He says, "This can be one hell of a frustrating process—you may have an overwhelming urge to throw in the towel and take up playing chess instead. One runner will swear on their Mother's grave that such-and-such a thing solved their problem, but their solution won't work at all for you." It cannot be overstressed, you must find what works for your feet.

8

The Components of Prevention

The one problem with our feet we most often experience, that drives us crazy, and costs us time and, in some cases, unfulfilled dreams—is blisters. These chapters on prevention deal with keeping our feet healthy by preventing the "dreaded" blisters.

Prevention works through a combination of components. Socks, powders, lubricants, skin tougheners, taping, orthotics, nutrition for the feet, proper hydration, anti-perspirants for the feet, gaiters, laces, and frequent sock and shoe changes are among the prevention components available to fix foot problems. You need to start with proper fitting shoes with a quality insole. No matter how good you tape, or how good your socks are, or how good any other component is, if the shoes fit incorrectly, you will have problems. Whatever you apply to your skin—powder, lubricant, or tape—must work together with anything surrounding your feet—the insoles, orthotics, socks, shoes, gaiters, and even your shoe laces—in order to prevent blisters. Cutting corners on any one of the factors can increase your chances of blistering.

Imagine a triangle with heat, friction, and moisture at its three sides. These three factors combine to make the skin more susceptible to blisters. Heat and moisture, in the presence of friction, lead to blisters.

Dr. David Hannaford, a podiatrist and runner, stresses that "If you eliminate any one of the three factors, you eliminate the blister." The triangle with these three factors, heat, friction, and moisture, sits on a base that has two levels.

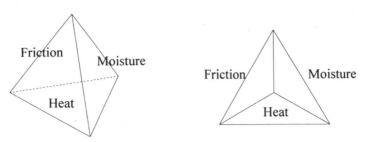

The three factors of blister formation

Each level of the base is a circle made up of components that can prevent these three factors from forming. Closest to the triangle is the top circle with the components of socks, powders, and lubricants—the first line of defense against blisters. Friction, which produces heat, can be reduced by wearing a sock with wicking properties, either alone or with an outer sock, or by using powders or lubricant. Moisture can be reduced with the wicking properties of certain socks and by using powders to keep the feet dry.

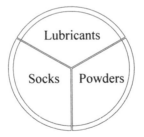

The top inner circle of blister prevention components

Socks are either single- or double-layer construction. Some single-layer socks, particularly those without wicking properties, allow friction to develop between the feet and the socks, which in turn can create blisters. Double-layer socks allow the sock layers to move against each other, which reduces friction between the feet and the first sock layer.

Powders reduce friction by reducing moisture on the skin that in turn reduces friction between the feet and the socks.

Lubricants create a shield, either greasy or non-greasy, to areas of the skin that are in contact during motion. This lubricant shield reduces chafing, which in turn reduces friction.

The bottom of the base is an outer circle made up of components that play a strong supporting role in prevention. This outer circle is made up of components including skin tougheners, taping, orthotics, nutrition for the feet and proper hydration, antiperspirants for the feet, gaiters, laces, and frequent sock and shoe changes. Each can contribute to the prevention of blisters and other problems. You could argue that these outer components should be identified as major components, and to some extent you may be right. Some components may be more important for your feet than for mine. The trick is to determine what we each need to keep our feet healthy under the stresses of our particular sport.

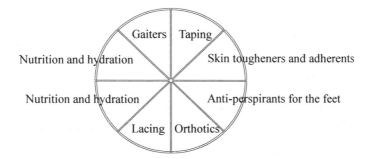

The bottom outer circle of blister prevention components

Skin tougheners form a coating to protect and toughen the skin. These products also help tape and blister patches adhere better to the skin.

Taping provides a barrier between the skin and socks so friction is reduced. Proper taping adds an extra layer of skin (the tape) to the foot to prevent hot spots and blisters. Taping can also be a treatment if hot spots and blisters do develop.

Orthotics help maintain the foot in a functionally neutral position so arch and pressure problems are relieved. Small pads for the feet may also help correct foot imbalances and pressure points. Nutrition for the feet includes creams and lotions so dry and callused feet are softened. The result is softer and smoother skin.

Proper hydration can help reduce swelling of the feet so the occurrence of hot spots and blisters is reduced.

Anti-perspirants for the feet helps those with sweaty feet by reducing the moisture that makes the feet more prone to blisters. Gaiters provide protection against dirt, rocks, and grit. These irritants cause friction and blisters as shoes and socks become dirty. Shoe and boot laces often cause friction or pressure problems. Adjusting laces can relieve this friction and pressure and make footwear more comfortable.

Frequent sock changes help keep the feet in good condition. Wet or moist socks can cause problems. Changing the socks also gives opportunity to reapply either powder or lubricant and deal with any hot spots before they become blisters. Sometimes shoes are also changed as they become overly dirty or wet.

Finding The Right Combination

Each runner and hiker needs to find what combination works for them. One may use Vaseline; another may use Zeasorb powder, while another may pre-tape his feet. They each may use one of many types and styles of socks. There are many combinations.

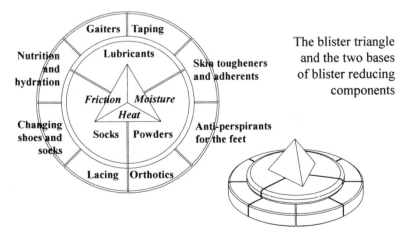

The blister triangle and the two bases of blister reducing components

Ultrarunner Dave Scott claims his feet are often "... as soft as a baby's bottom" after the 100-mile Western States Endurance

Run. Dave has found that he rarely gets foot problems. He trims his toenails, uses a small amount of Vaseline, and regularly changes his shoes and socks. That is what works for him. At the other extreme is the runner who has the skin falling off his feet from midsoles to heels. One hiker may end a six-day hike having had a few simple foot problems while another may have suffered with major problems the whole trip. Determine what foot problems you normally experience, study this book, and then begin the task of finding what works best for your feet.

Ultrarunner Tim Twietmeyer has won the grueling 100-mile Western States Endurance Run four times while accumulating 17 silver belt buckles for sub-24 hour finishes. Over the past five years, in addition to running ultras, he has enjoyed fastpacking in the California High Sierras. He has found the differences interesting.

A week before running a 100-mile trail ultra Tim trims his toenails as short as possible. The morning of the run he coats his feet with lanolin to reduce friction, provide warmth if running in snow or through water, and make his skin more resilient to getting all wrinkled. Then he pulls on a pair of Thorlo Ultrathin socks. His strategy is "... that the more sock you wear, the more moisture close to the foot. The more moisture the more blisters and skin problems." He usually wears the same pair of shoes and socks the entire way. Tim acknowledges "... my feet don't usually have problems, and when they do, I'm close enough to the end to gut it out."

Tim has found that fastpacking affects his feet differently. When he did the John Muir Trail in 1992 (five days and ten hours to do 210 miles), his feet were trashed more than ever before. His group of five experienced ultrarunners averaged 14 hours per day on the rough trail. Tim remembers, "We covered the ground so fast that my feet swelled and I almost couldn't get my shoes on the last day." He used the same strategy of lanolin and thin socks. Instead of running shoes he chose lightweight hiking boots. Foot repair became the group's daily ritual as the 40-mile days took their toll. They realized that "... an important strategy for keeping our feet from getting any worse was to get that first piece of duct tape on in just the right spot and making it stick. If we did that, our feet held up pretty well." By the end of the fifth day the last piece of duct tape had been used on their feet. Tim's cardinal rule for fastpacking is to "Keep your feet dry." While that can be hard to do when fighting afternoon thunderstorms, if your feet are wet too long, it's only a matter of time before they blister. Whether running ultras or fastpacking, Tim knows the importance of keeping his feet healthy and has experimented to find what works well for his feet.

In experimenting to find what works for your feet, be creative. There are many unique ways to save your feet. Clive Saffery ran the extreme Badwater, Death Valley, to Mt. Whitney ultramarathon and came up with a creative method of protecting his feet from the heat. In the 1999 Badwater race he took an additional precaution to his usual regimen of tapering, and use of Vaseline and powder. In order to reduce heat on his feet he duct taped a cut up space blanket on all the non white parts of his shoe uppers and lined the under side of his shoe insoles in the same way, using small pieces of duct tape to hold the silver blanket on the shoe and insole. Apart from one small heel blister at 122 miles he was trouble free the whole race in spite of the temperatures. The space blanket under his shoe insoles fared worse however—when it was removed after climbing out of Death Valley it had been reduced to a transparent piece of cling film! It had certainly done its' job though.

We need to understand the importance of other elements that contribute to prevention. These elements are discussed in *Part Three: Treatments* of this book. Proper strength training and conditioning will help make the foot and ankle stronger and more resistant to sprains and strains. Good care of the skin will help prevent calluses. Quality insoles and orthotics can help prevent or relieve the problems of plantar fasciitis, Achilles tendinitis, heel pain, metatarsalgia, Morton's neuroma, Morton's foot, sesamoiditis, corns, and bunions. Good-fitting footwear will help prevent problems with toenails, arches, and blisters. In short, everything you put on or around your foot becomes related to how well your foot functions.

9

Socks

Socks perform four basic functions: cushioning, protection, warmth, and absorbing moisture off the skin. The sock fabric and weave will determine how well they do in each of the four areas. Socks made from synthetic fabrics wick moisture away from the skin and through the sock to its outer surface where it can evaporate.

Some athletes wear the common cotton crew sock while others swear by synthetic socks or synthetic double layer socks. Each method has its reasons. If cotton crew socks work for you, continue using them. If however, hot spots and/or blisters plague you, consider trying other types of socks. Cotton tube socks should always be avoided for both running and hiking because of their loose fit. Some have discovered socks with individual toes and like these because they avoid the typical problems when dirt and grime would collect between the toes and cause friction.

For my first 24-hour track run I wore thick cotton socks and used gobs of Vaseline on my feet. That was what everyone else seemed to be doing, so that was what I did. It didn't take long for blisters to develop on my heels and toes that reduced me to a slow walk. Even so, I managed to get in a respectable 103 miles. Without the early foot problems, I am sure I could have done another ten miles. I learned the hard way what did not work on my feet and set out to find what did work.

Not everyone needs a primer on how to put on your socks, but it is important to know a few tricks. Seems like a simple thing but it can make the difference between sore, blistered feet and happy feet. Rick Schick suggests to, "First be sure your socks are clean and free of debris. Hold them by the cuff, pull them through the closed fist of the other hand and then whip them in the air a couple times. Turn them inside out and then repeat. If the socks have a heavy seam at the toe, wear them inside out. Next massage your feet and between the toes making sure there is absolutely no grit or other debris. Then either roll or bunch the socks up so the toes can be placed in the toe of the sock. Be sure the seam is across the top of the toes and if possible not lap around the small toe. Now bring the sock up over the rest of the foot and up the leg, use a massaging motion to be sure there are no wrinkles and to detect any rough spots or debris.

Next, remove the insert from your shoe and inspect it. Remove any lint, toe jam, or other debris. Now bang the shoes together sole to sole a couple times and then tap the heel on the ground. Now shake out any debris and reach inside and feel all surfaces for debris or other problems. Replace the inserts and put on your shoes. Sounds complicated but the whole process takes less than a minute and can prevent many foot problems."

Clean socks can feel heavenly. When hiking, wash yesterday's socks and let them dry on the back of your pack. Try to change socks several times during a 100-mile run and once during a 50-mile run. During multi-day events, try to change socks several times a day. If clean socks are unavailable from your crew, try to wash the dirty socks so they are clean for later use.

You may be one of a growing number of athletes who wear socks inside out. Rob Langsdorf recommends simply turning your socks inside out to help prevent blisters, "Most socks have a rib near the toe where the sock is pulled together. The manufactures put this on the inside of the sock, so it looks nice. Unfortunately it tends to rub the tops and sides of the toes and can cause blisters."

Types of Socks

Socks come in a variety of fabrics: cotton, cotton blends, synthetics, silk, wool and wool blends, and fleece. An overview of these

materials provides insights into their uses. Read the product information on the sock's packaging and try several types to find those
that work best for you.

- **Cotton**   A 100% cotton sock provides no wicking or insulating properties and therefore moisture is retained against
  the skin. In damp or wet cotton, your feet are generally wet,
  cold, and more prone to blistering.
- **Cotton blends**   A cotton blend, with cotton as the main
  product, offers a limited advantage over a pure cotton sock.
  Cotton may be blended with Lycra, nylon, rayon, and acrylic.
- **Fleece**   Fleece socks are soft, provide exceptional warmth,
  and dry faster than wool.
- **Synthetics**   The newer synthetic material socks offer
  protection against blisters caused by moisture, poor fit, hot
  spots, slippage, or friction. These are made of hydrophobic
  materials, which means they don't like moisture or water.
  Moisture-wicking fabrics like Capilene, Coolmax, Olefin, or
  polypropylene wick moisture and perspiration away from the
  skin to the outer layer of the sock. Synthetic insulators like
  Hollofil, Thermax, or Thermastat help provide insulation.
  Some of these socks are single layer while others are double
  layer. Most of the socks use one of the above fabrics blended
  with cotton, nylon, Lycra spandex, or acrylic.
- **Silk**   Silk socks are slick and generally used as liners.
  With low wicking properties and low heat retention they do
  not dry as fast as the newer synthetics.
- **Wool**   Wool wicks while retaining its cushioning but can
  be scratchy and rough.
- **Wool blends**   Wool blends make for a more comfortable fit and a tougher-wearing sock. Socks made from worsted wool are soft and durable. Merino wool, from sheep with
  a lighter and softer coat, is less resilient but very soft and
  comfortable. Wool may also be blended with other fabrics.

Technology is moving faster than we can keep up—even in
socks. A new sock uses a patented "Blister Guard" technology
utilizing DuPont's Teflon Fiber as a low friction fiber that come in

contact with the skin to prevent hot spots that cause blisters, abrasions, and calluses. These socks have passed strenuous tests by achieving an 80% to 100% reduction of blisters in cases where the previous occurrence was 100% blistering. Teflon fibers are woven into the fabric of the sock at the toes, forefoot, and the heels. After over 50 washings, there was almost 0% loss of the Teflon fibers. The socks are being marketed by various sock companies with combinations of traditional fibers such as acrylic, wool, nylon, and polyester, as well as performance fibers such as Coolmax and Lycra. Look for the Blister Guard symbol when you buy your next pair of socks. The sock's packaging offers an unconditional guarantee for no hot spots, no blisters, and no calluses! John Prohira recalls, "I thought that blisters were a fact of life or dues to be paid." Then he was given a pair of Blister Guard socks by a friend and wore them on an 11-hour run with no hot spots or blisters.

The weave of the sock will vary depending on the material. Socks will range from a loose weave to a dense weave. The loose weave will feel coarse and provide less insulation. The dense weave will feel softer and generally offers more cushioning. Put your hand inside a sock and stretch the foot portion with your fingers to see the weave. Denser-weave socks will show less space between the fibers.

Double-layer socks are used to help reduce or eliminate the likelihood of blisters developing. The two layers moving against each other instead of against the skin reduces skin friction. Most double-layer socks utilize wicking properties to move moisture away from the feet. Before wearing any double-layer sock, align the layers with your hand and then roll the socks on the foot for the best fit.

Buy socks that fit your feet. The heels, toes, and length should fit snugly without sagging or being stretched too tight. Socks that are too big will bunch up and cause friction and skin irritation. Socks that are too small can cause the toes and joints to rub harder against the socks. Turn them inside out and look at the toe seams. Avoid those with bulky seams because they can rub, causing hot spots and blisters. After buying socks be sure to try them on with your shoes or boots to be sure they fit together and are not too tight. Remember also to discard socks when they become thread-bare and too thin to provide their advertised benefits. The heels of your socks are a good indicator of the amount of padding and loft.

Sock garters can prevent socks from slipping and getting wrinkled inside of the shoe causing blisters and hot spots. This is especially true when feet are wet either from rain, stream cross-ings or excessive perspiration. It also is more of a problem on trails with steep climbs and descents although it can happen when on dry level surfaces. Making a sock garter can prevent it. Go to a craft store or sewing supply center and buy a couple feet of inch and a quarter elastic used in pants etc. Be sure to get the ribbed or "roll proof" variety. Measure around your leg at the narrowest point, just above the ankle, and then make a loop of the elastic about one half inch shorter. When placed over the sock at that point the gar ter should feel snug but not tight.

Many stores offer a basket of socks to use when trying on shoes and boots. Try to avoid these and instead use your own socks when shopping. This way you get to feel the fit with your personal socks and avoid picking up a foot fungus from another shopper.

The following sections identify specific *Running Socks*, *Hik-ing Socks*, *Sock Liners*, *High-Technology Socks*, and *Sandal Socks*. Review each of these sections for an overview of the wide range of available socks. Many of the socks may be used for running, hiking, and adventure racing. Check them out at a store near you to feel them and read their packaging information.

Running Socks

The following are a sampling of running socks typically available in running stores. Check your local store for the types they carry. If the store does not stock the types described here, or those you have seen in a magazine, ask the staff if they can order other types.

The following list of sock companies is provided to show how diverse the field is and how many different types of socks there are to choose from. There are also many more companies not listed. Each company introduces new versions of their socks each year. As an example, one company that makes running socks, Bridgedale, in a recent brochure, offers four types of sandal socks, nine types of running/walking socks, 12 types of hiking socks, and the list goes on. New fabrics and combinations of fabrics make the sock selection ever changing. Your local stores will have displays of many of these socks or check out the web sites listed. Investigate your sock options and talk to others about their preferences to determine which socks may be best for your hiking needs.

Products

BaySix   BaySix offers either single- or double-layer socks in ankle and crew lengths. Their Wonderspun yarns made from rayon wrapped in nylon provide wicking properties that transfer heat and moisture away from the foot. The double-layer sock is designed to allow the layers to move against each other, reducing the friction against the skin. For more information contact BaySix, 1408 Christian Avenue, Durham, NC 27705; (888) baysix1; www.baysix.com.

Fox River Fox River makes a Coolmax triathlon sock. For more information contact Fox River, PO Box 298, Osage, IA 50461; (888) 288-2431.

Ridgeview   Ridgeview offers crew and ankle-high socks of a Coolmax, stretch nylon, and elastic combination.

Runique   AA-R Hosiery makes the original double-layer sock from Wonderspun yarns with stretch nylon and spandex. For more information contact AA-R Hosiery, PO Box 1118, Elon College, NC 27244.

SmartWool   SmartWool socks from Duke Designs are made from very soft Merino wool and Lycra and use their Active-Fit system. These wool socks do not itch and provide good wicking action while keeping your feet warm in the winter and cool in the summer. For more information contact Smartwool, (800) 550-9665; www.smartwool.com.

Spenco Multi-Fresh   Spenco uses acrylic Amicor Plus yarn embedded with anti-bacterial and anti-fungal agents to keep feet fresh and comfortable. With a reinforced heel and toe for ex-

tra durability and cushioning, a support weave in the arch and forefoot, fiction is reduced and fit improved. For more information
contact Spenco Medical Corporation, PO Box 2501, Waco, TX
76702-2501; (800) 877-3626; www.spenco.com.

Thorlo   Thorlo uses their Thorlo System Fit to make socks
for specific sports activities. The combination of acrylic and stretch
nylon helps to reduce blisters and other foot discomforts. The socks
have a combination of resilient, spongy pads at the ball and heel
and a lower-density pad at the arch for a contour fit and reduction
in bulk. The socks use Foot Health yarns to wick moisture away
from the foot. Choose between highly cushioned or thinner, lightweight socks. For more information contact Thorlo, Inc., PO Box
5399, Statesville, NC 28687-5399; (800) 438-0286;
www.thorlo.com.

Wigwam   Wigwam offers a complete line of socks for specific sports activities: running, triathlons, cycling, etc. Their
Ultimax sock line uses Olefin, a moisture-absorbing acrylic, nylon, and Lycra spandex. Another style uses a combination of
Coolmax, cotton, and stretch nylon. For more information contact
Wigwam Mills Inc., PO Box 818, Sheboygan, WI 53082-0818;
(800) 558-7760

Wrightsock   Wrightsock offers a double-layer sock
made of nylon and Coolmax. The two layers move against each
other to reduce the friction against the skin. For more information
contact WrightSock, (800) 654-7191.

Other Sock Options   Other types of sock and combinations of socks that have been tried include:

- Will Uher likes rock climber's socks that are thin and fit snugly
  on his feet.
- Any two pairs of socks can be used together, as an inner and
  outer layer. Usually, the thinner layer is worn inside.
- Ankle-high nylons. Yes, nylons—as an inner sock! Sid Snyder
  found that by wearing ankle high nylons under his Thorlo
  socks he does not get blisters. No tape and no Vaseline—just
  the nylons. He had blistered so bad on another long trail event
  that he was on crutches for three days and knew he had to try

something new. Be sure to try this combination before a competitive event. Try them with the sock you normally wear, preferably a wicking sock. When using nylons for trail running or hiking, be sure to try them on uphills and downhills since some individuals may be bothered by the slippery smooth nylon.

• Camping stores carry socks that can be used for running. New socks are continually being designed. Acorn makes a fleece Tekna-Sport sock with excellent moisture management. Dahlgren offers a Dri-Stride Trail Fitness sock with moisture management zones. Smartwool makes an Ultra Thin soft merino wool and nylon moisture wicking sock.

Hiking Socks

Hiking socks are different from running socks. Hikers most often wear crew or high-top socks. Some wear a wool outer sock with a liner that has wicking properties. Hikers could also try the thinner double-layer wicking socks in a crew top style. These wear well, wick moisture away, and are made to reduce the possibility of blisters.

Pacific Crest Trail hiker Matthew Jankowicz used to get blisters, especially on long hikes over 20 miles a day. He tried tape, moleskin, and different kinds of boots. Finally, he switched to wearing three pair of socks and it worked. He uses one pair of wicking socks over which he wears two pair of boot socks. Matthew says, "I know some people think I'm crazy but it works very well for me and I have hiked thousands of miles this way without getting any blisters on my feet." Another hiker, going by the trail name of Morning Glory, found that wearing a thin liner sock, a Thorlo sock, and finally a wool-blend hiking sock worked well. She bought boots that would take the three pairs of socks. If wearing heavy socks for winter, wear a shoe a half size larger than normal. If you wear your normal size shoe it compresses the heavy sock and at best you gain little in the way of insulation. In the worst case it is so tight in inhibits blood flow to the toes and results in frostbite.

The following list of sock companies is provided to show how diverse the field is and how many different types of socks there are to choose from. There are also many more companies not listed. Each company introduces new versions of their socks each year. As an example, one company, Bridgedale, in a recent brochure, offers four types of sandal socks, nine types of running/walking socks, 12 types of hiking socks, and the list goes on. New fabrics and combinations of fabrics make the sock selection ever changing. Your camping and backpacking store will have displays of many of these socks, or check out the sock company's web sites. Investigate your sock options and talk to others about their preferences to determine which socks may be best for your hiking needs.

Products

Acorn Fleece Socks   Acorn Products make fleece socks that can be used for hiking. Made with Polartec fleece fabric these socks provide lightweight warmth and rapid drying. For more information contact Acorn, 2 Cedar Street, Lewiston, ME 04243; (800) USA-CORN.

Bridgedale   Fabric combinations may include Coolmax, cotton, nylon, wool, or Lycra spandex. For information contact Bridgedale, PO Box 12278, Everett, WA 98206; (888) 79-SOCKS; www.bridgedale.co.uk.

Dahlgren   Dahlgren Footwear makes Dri-Stride socks with their Climate Knit system. The socks have Patented Zones of wool, cotton, and Dursaspun Smart Yarns to control temperature and provide wicking of moisture. For more information contact Dahlgren Footwear Inc., PO Box 660614, Arcadia, CA 91066; (800) 635-8539; www.dahlgrenfootwear.com.

Fox River   Fox River socks are made with their Wick Dry system. Individual sock fabrics include combinations of acrylic, Coolmax, stretch nylon, worsted wool, cotton, or polypropylene. For more information contact Fox River, PO Box 298, Osage, IA 50461; (888) 288-2431.

Patagonia   Patagonia offers socks with their soft, quick drying, and moisture wicking Capilene. Fabric combinations include Capilene, worsted wool, and stretch nylon. For more information contact Patagonia Inc., 800-336-9090.

REI   REI makes a complete line of socks with their label. Individual sock fabrics include combinations of acrylic, stretch nylon, worsted wool, cotton, Lycra spandex, or polypropylene. For more information contact REI, 1700 45th Street East, Sumner, WA 98390; (800) 426-4840; http://www.rei.com.

SmartWool   SmartWool socks from Duke Designs are made from very soft Merino wool and Lycra and use their Active-Fit system. These wool socks do not itch and provide good wicking action while keeping your feet warm in the winter and cool in the summer. For more information contact For more information contact Smartwool, (800) 550-9665; www.smartwool.com.

Spenco Multi-Fresh   Spenco uses acrylic Amicor Plus yarn embedded with anti-bacterial and anti-fungal agents to keep feet fresh and comfortable. With a reinforced heel and toe for extra durability and cushioning, a support weave in the arch and forefoot, fiction is reduced and fit improved. For more information contact Spenco Medical Corporation, PO Box 2501, Waco, TX 76702-2501; (800) 877-3626; www.spenco.com.

Thermohair   Thermohair makes fuzzy socks from the fleece of the Turkish Angora goats, adding 25% nylon for stretch. Incredibly soft with their cushy knitted loops, they do not itch. These socks provide great warmth while also wicking moisture from the skin. They are long-lasting and very durable. Available in regular sock height and low styles. For more information contact Thermohair, PO Box 213, South Mountain, Ontario, Canada, K0E 1W0; (877) 766-4247; www.thermohair.com.

Thorlo   Thorlo uses their Thorlo System Fit to make socks for specific sports activities. The socks are made from a combination of fabrics and each may include acrylic, Coolmax, stretch nylon, Lycra spandex, or wool. For more information contact Thorlo, Inc., PO Box 5399, Statesville, NC 28687-5399; (800) 438-0286; www.thorlo.com.

Wigwam   Wigwam offers a complete line of socks for hiking, many with their Wonder-Wick Foot Drying System.

Individual sock fabrics include combinations of acrylic, Olefin, Hollofil polyester, Coolmax, stretch nylon, wool, cotton, polypropylene, or Lycra. For more information contact Wigwam Mills Inc., PO Box 818, Sheboygan, WI 53082-0818; (800) 558-7760.

Sock Liners

Sock liners are thin, smooth, and are usually worn under a heavier insulating or cushioning sock, typically wool. Most liner are made from hydrophobic fibers to wick moisture away from the foot and into the outer sock and are lightweight and quick drying. A liner will perform with the outer sock the same as the double layer socks. Friction will occur between the two layers and not against the skin, reducing the chance of blisters. When shopping for liners, look for a style with wicking properties. While many runners are converting to the double-layer socks, some still prefer a two-sock system using liners.

Products

Fox River   Fox River Wick & Dry Sockliner are made from polypropylene. For more information contact Fox River, PO Box 298, Osage, IA 50461; (888) 288-2431.

Helly-Hansen   Helly-Hansen Polypro Liners are made with polypropylene and are available in several thicknesses that offer options in use with outer socks.

Patagonia   Patagonia's liner socks are durable, thin, and fast-drying, made from Capilene polyester and stretch nylon. For more information contact Patagonia Inc., 800-336-9090.

SmartWool   SmartWool socks from Duke Designs are made from very soft Merino wool and Lycra and use their Active-Fit system. These wool socks do not itch and provide good wicking action while keeping your feet warm in the winter and cool in the summer. They make one liner sock. For more information contact For more information contact Smartwool, (800) 550-9665;

www.smartwool.com.

Wigwam   Wigwam offers several sock liners. One style is made with the Thermastat Wonder-Wick Foot Dry System to protect feet against cold and blisters. Other styles use Coolmax, polypropylene, Chinese Silk and nylon, or a combination of worsted wool, stretch nylon, and Lycra spandex. For more information contact Wigwam Mills Inc., PO Box 818, Sheboygan, WI 53082-0818; (800) 558-7760.

Z-Dry One   Z Knit makes a liner sock made from polypropylene and nylon. For more information contact Z Knit, Niota, TN 37826.

High-Technology Oversocks

Oversocks are special high-technology socks that combine waterproof technology and the comfort of traditional socks into a somewhat baggy-looking sock. They were developed for anyone who participates in outdoor activities where the feet are exposed to water. Widely used by hunters and fishermen, they are being discovered by runners, hikers, and adventure racers. Feet are kept dry and comfortable even though the shoes or boots may be soaked and muddy.

National champion ultrarunner Roy Pirrung tested the high technology oversock SealSkinz for a year in all kinds of weather. Roy recalls his win at the 100-KM Glacial Trail Run, a grueling race through the wet Kettle Moraine State Forest in Wisconsin. "It had rained the day before and conditions were sloppy. As other runners stopped every 10 miles to change their wet socks, I just raced ahead. I ended up finishing the race within 25 seconds of the course record, and without any blisters." In wet and cold conditions, oversocks can work wonders. Roy found that SealSkinz have helped him to train outside in minus 25-degree weather with a wind-chill factor of minus 80. His feet "... stayed warm, dry and comfortable."

Oversocks work best when used with a Coolmax or other wicking material sock liner. This further enhances moisture dispersion as well as comfort. Care must be taken when pulling the socks on or off to avoid tearing the inner membrane. A torn membrane will allow water to penetrate at the tear site.

Ideally, oversocks should not be submersed in water over the cuffs. If the cuff is loose fitting, water may get inside the sock. Once water has gone down the leg into the sock, the wicking process slows or stops, depending on the amount of water in the sock. Over time, the body's heat combined with the wicking action of the Coolmax liner may dry the inside of the socks, but this depends on both the amount of water inside the sock and the degree of activity. Roy recommends wearing tights over the cuffs to provide a covering seal.

An alternative to these type socks is to put on a pair of thick socks, then a soft plastic bag over the feet, finally adding a thin outer sock. The inner socks, in the plastic bags, will get damp from body sweat and heat, but will stay reasonably comfortable compared to totally wet feet. The plastic bags that bread comes in work well, but check them first for leaks by blowing in them and squeezing them lightly while holding them closed.

Products

REI/Gore-Tex Oversocks   REI/Gore-Tex Oversocks are waterproof, breathable and designed to be worn over a pair of thin wicking socks. The socks have a Gore-Tex membrane laminated between inner and outer fabric layers. The inner seams are sealed with Gore Seam tape. The sole and back panel is made of a non-stretch Gore-Tex fabric to increase durability and prevent slippage. The upper panels are stretchable Gore-Tex fabrics for flexibility and conformity to the foot's shape. A spandex cuff helps the socks stay up. When wearing these socks, watch for skin irritations caused by the inner seams. These socks are available through all REI stores or through REI mail order. For more information contact REI, 1700 45th Street East, Sumner, WA 98390; (800) 426-4840; www.rei.com.

SealSkinz Waterproof MVT Socks   SealSkinz socks from Dupont are seamless waterproof socks that use moisture vapor transpiration (MVT) technology. The socks are made in a thin, lightweight, three-layer design. An inner Coolmax or Thermastat liner wicks moisture away from the skin while a middle layer of vapor-permeable membrane allows perspiration to escape and prevents water from entering. The outer layer uses nylon for abrasion resistance and durability. The Lycra spandex cuff ensures the socks will stay up. Their seamless design gives them a positive edge in preventing blisters.

The All-Season Socks are made for general wear and use Coolmax as a wicking liner. The Insulated Socks are made for cold conditions to protect feet from extreme temperatures and use Thermastat as a liner to both wick away moisture and retain body heat. An Over-the-Calf sock is also available. An All-Sport version in ankle and crew lengths is perfect for runners. The socks are made in small, medium, large and extra large. SealSkinz can be ordered through sporting good stores and outdoor specialty stores. Contact Dupont for the dealer nearest you. For more information contact Dupont, c/o GS&F, 1002 Industrial Road, Old Hickory, TN 37138-3693; (800) 868-2629; www.sealskinz.com.

Many of the Eco-Challenge Adventure Race teams use SealSkinz socks to keep their feet free of blisters, abrasions caused by dirt and grime, and the effects of water immersion during their long, multi-day competition.

Seirus Neo-Sock and StormSock   Seirus Neo-Socks provides warmth from closed-cell insulation for winter activities. It is made from four-way stretch neoprene with breathable macro porous technology to prevent moisture buildup while sealing in body heat. These socks have a nylon fabric on either side of the neoprene that allows moisture to pass through. The StormSock has an outer layer of Lycra, an inner membrane of high-technology Weather Shield that stops wind and water, and is lined with Polartec fleece. Both socks have seams that should be checked for waterproofing. For more information contact Seirus Innovative Accessories, 9076 Carroll Way, San Diego, CA 92121; (800) 447-3787.

Sandal Socks

The advent of newer and better designs of sport sandals makes them popular for general wear. Some of the better styles can be used for running or hiking. Multi-day hikers can wear sandals in camp as a refreshing change from their heavier hiking boots. While regular socks can be worn with sandals, specific sandal socks are offered.

Products

Acorn   Acorn Products make a fleece for lightweight warmth and rapid drying. For more information contact Acorn, 2 Cedar Street, Lewiston, ME 04243; (800) USA-CORN.

Bridgedale   Bridgedale makes two socks for sandals. One is made from Coolmax, combed cotton, nylon, and Lycra. The other is made from combed cotton, nylon, and Lycra. For information contact Bridgedale, PO Box 12278, Everett, WA 98206; (888) 79-SOCKS; www.bridgedale.co.uk.

Thermohair   Thermohair makes fuzzy socks from the fleece of the Turkish Angora goats, adding 25% nylon for stretch. Incredibly soft with their cushy knitted loops, they do not itch. These socks provide great warmth while also wicking moisture from the skin. They are long-lasting and very durable. Available in regular sock height and low styles. For more information contact Thermohair, PO Box 213, South Mountain, Ontario, Canada, K0E 1W0; (877) 766-4247; www.thermohair.com.

Wyoming Wear   Wyoming Wear makes several sandal socks than can also be used for hiking. Made from fleece, these retain warmth. For more information contact Wyoming Wear, PO Box 3127, Jackson Hole, WY 83001; (800) WYO-WEAR; www.wyomingwear.com.

The Option of Not Wearing Socks

In 1973 a running magazine advertised "New, lean, and luxurious—the first sockless athletic shoe." After three years of development, Bare Foot Gear, offered the "Original Sockless Shoe" with prime leather inside and out, no staples or nails, no seams or ridges, and no textiles to touch your foot. Just unpainted and unsealed leather. Cupping the foot only at the heel and instep, it offered a large space up front for flexion and good air circulation. It claimed that with a drier foot, friction is minimized. Looking at the ad today, we might find humor in the ad's statement "Most men prefer no socks because of the sheer maleness of the feel."

There is the option, like the shoe designers hoped people would buy into, of not wearing socks. Some prefer this option. Matt Mahoney found that for him, the best way to prevent blisters was to train for them. Walking barefoot and sometimes running barefoot on grass, dirt, or sand toughened the skin on his feet. He does not wear socks with shoes, but rotates between several brands of shoes to develop calluses at every spot that could rub. Matt found that socks caused his feet to slide around inside his shoes and he couldn't grip the trail on steep hills. When he finds spots rubbing, he uses tape, Vaseline, or Blister Relief.

This type of barefoot running or running in shoes without socks takes time and careful monitoring of your feet to avoid problems. Matt has conditioned his feet by walking a mile barefoot on roads every day. He estimates he runs 15% of the time barefoot on grass and dirt and the other 85% in shoes without socks. He has strengthened the small muscles and tendons in his feet. The skin on the bottom of his feet has toughened to provide some degree of protection for running barefoot. Gradually toughen your feet with short periods of barefoot walking before trying to run barefoot. If trying to go without socks, check your shoes for rough seams or ridges that can cut into your feet. Like Matt, use tape or a lubricant on areas that rub. Matt strongly believes we need to, "Learn to run in simple shoes, sandals, or barefoot as people have done for thousands of years before Nike." Barefoot running and hiking is becoming more accepted. The section *Sandals* on page 37 gives information on sandals for walking, running, and hiking.

Walking and running barefoot can be an excellent way to condition your feet in order to prevent blisters when you do wear boots or shoes. Your skin will be tougher and you may develop calluses. Yet, be forewarned—this is no guarantee that you will not get blisters! Kevin Sayers had feet that were a "... bushman/ firewalker's dream, impervious to almost all minor punctures and discomfort." Yet he would get blisters underneath his calluses on the balls of his feet. He learned that he would rather tape a blister that he could see rather than one that's beneath the skin. Blisters under skin-toughened calluses can take four to six weeks to heal instead of the usual two weeks it takes a normal blister to heal.

Lest you think that going barefoot is only for walking and runners, consider the group called Barefoot Hikers. Barefoot Chris, using his trail name, a member of Barefoot Hikers of PA-NJ-DE-MD, recalls the shocked reaction of hikers they encountered while on a weeklong barefoot backpacking trip on the Appalachian Trail. They heard stories of many other barefoot hikers, including at least two that had done the entire trail without shoes. The web site www.barefooters.org/hikers has more information on hiking barefoot. The book *The Barefoot Hiker* by Richard Frazine is about hiking barefoot.

10

Powders

There are powders and then there are powders. Cornstarch and talcum powder have been used for years as foot powders, but times and powders have changed. Having tried a super absorbent powder, I would never again use a plain powder. Powders can be effective in reducing moisture on the feet. Their effectiveness depends on their ability to absorb moisture while not caking into clumps. Clumps can cause skin irritations and blisters. When using powders, remember to reapply the powder at regular intervals or after the feet have been exposed to water. If you have problems with athlete's foot or other skin problems, use a medicated powder.

After lightly powdering your feet, massage the powder between the toes. Then roll your socks on to the level of the heel and put some powder in the socks. Then squeeze off the top of the sock and shake your foot and repeatedly shake the sock until powder comes through the sock.

Hiker and ultrarunner Randy Gehrke tried powders with great success. He regularly powders his feet and changes his socks in 100-mile runs. In his last two 100-mile trail runs he has not had any problem with his feet.

Products

Cornstarch   An inexpensive foot powder, cornstarch, can be found at your local supermarket. It works as an absorbent. One method of application is to fill a plastic Ziplock bag with a handful of cornstarch. Shake the bag around your foot to coat all surfaces of the foot and then put on a clean, dry pair of socks.

Gold Bond   Gold Bond is a medicated body powder that contains active ingredient zinc oxide as a skin protector and menthol to cool and relieve itching. Use the extra-strength powder for maximum benefits in absorbing excessive moisture. Gold Bond is made by Chattem, Inc. and is available through your local drug store and pharmacy.

Bromi-Talc   Gordon Laboratories makes Bromi-Talc, a triple action foot powder. Bromi-Talc contains potassium alum, an astringent that retards perspiration; bentonite, a highly absorbent agent; and the highest-grade talc powder for absorption. Bromi-Talc Plus powder contains additional properties to control excessive foot odor. Available only by special order through your local drug store, pharmacy, or podiatrist from Gordon Laboratories, 6801 Ludlow Street, Upper Darby, PA 19082; (800) 356-7870.

Odor-Eater's Foot Powder   Odor-Eater's packaging lists this foot powder as 25 time more absorbent than talc. It is typically found in most drug stores and pharmacies.

Zeasorb   The success of Zeasorb is in its super absorbent powder, which absorbs almost four times more moisture than plain talcum powder. Zeasorb contains talc, a highly absorbent polymer-carbohydrate acrylic copolymer, and microporous cellulose for super absorbency. This powder is very efficient and works without caking. The talc provides softness and lubrication to reduce friction and heat buildup. Their second powder, ZeasorbAF, with miconazole nitrate 2%, provides broad antifungal therapy and moisture control. Look for it at drug stores or order it through your local pharmacy. For more information contact Stiefel Laboratories, Inc., 255 Alhambra Circle, Coral Gables, FL 33134-7412; (305) 443-3800.

11

Lubricants

Like powders, there are lubricants and then there are lubricants. Two of the old time tried-and-true lubricants are Lanolin and Vaseline. However technology has led to new formulas. Many runners have discovered Bag Balm or Udder Balm. Others make their own special formulas.

Robert Boeder used Andrew Lovy's formula on his feet in 1994 when he completed the Grand Slam of trail ultrarunning, running four 100-mile runs in 14 weeks. Robert comments that, "The idea is that these lotional charms will have the desired magical effect and blisters will not arise from my feet during the race."[11] This formula worked well for him. Since that time he switched to Bag Balm and then back to Vaseline, mainly because of its availability. Jim Benike found success using Udder Balm on his feet and then wearing socks to bed. He used Udder Balm more as a skin softener and conditioner than as a lubricant. Udder creams may go by different names, i.e., Bag Balm, Udder Balm, Dr. Naylor's Udder Balm, Aunt Irma's Udder Balm, etc.

Studies have shown that lubricants may initially reduce friction but over long periods of time they may actually increase friction. After one hour the friction levels returned to their baseline factor and after three hours the friction levels were 35% above the baseline. As the lubricants are absorbed into the skin and into the socks, friction returns and increases.[12] What we must learn from this is the need to reapply lubricants at frequent intervals.

Use lubricants on your feet, hands, underarms, inner thighs, and nipples—anywhere you chafe. The important thing to remember about lubricants is to clean the old off before applying a new coating. This is especially true during trail runs and hiking when dust and dirt buildup can foul the lubricant with grit. Wipe off the old stuff with a cleansing towelette or an alcohol wipe.

As always, try any new product before using it in a competitive event or taking it on a long hike. It is foolhardy to buy something and count on it in competition or on a six-day hike without trying it first. It may not work for you. Try any lubricant on a small patch of skin to be sure you are not allergic to the ingredients.

Products

Andrew Lovy's Formula   Andrew Lovy, in an article "New Blister Formula Revealed! Free!,"[13] shared a formula which he developed over several years. It has helped him solve his blister and friction problems. Take A and D Ointment, Vaseline, and Desitin ointment and mix together equal amounts. To this add Vitamin E cream and Aloe Vera cream (the thickness can be varied by the amount of these two ingredients). The result is a salve. For a thinner mixture, use Vitamin E and Aloe Vera ointment instead of the creams. Andrew recommends that the evening before your run, apply a thin layer to clean skin where friction occurs. In the morning, before you run, apply a more generous amount to friction areas. Add more to problem areas as necessary during the run. Shop around to find the ingredients in sizes appropriate for the total amount you want to mix.

Avon Silicone Glove   Avon makes this silicone cream for hands but it works equally well on feet. Its non-greasy and non-sticky formula lubricates while protecting against dryness and irritants as it softens. It is available in a handy 1.5-ounce tube. For more information contact Avon Products, 9 West 57th Street, NY, NY 10019; (800) FOR-AVON

Bag Balm   Bag Balm comes in a green tin which has become familiar to many runners. While Bag Balm is made and advertised for use on cow udders, it has found acceptance in sports circles. Consisting of a combination of lanolin, petrolatum, 8-hydroxy, and quinoline sulfate, many have found the salve to offer healing properties. It can be used on cracked, callused, or sore skin, or simply as a lubricant for your feet or other body areas. Available in one- or 10-ounce tins, it is usually found in feed stores and tack shops, but is becoming easier to find in many drug stores and hardware stores. For more information contact the Dairy Association Co. (East of the Rockies) PO Box 145, Lyndonville, VT 05851; (800) 232-3610; or Smith Sales Service (West of the Rockies), 16372 SW 72nd Avenue, Portland, OR 97223; (503) 639-5479; www.bagbalm.com (no online sales)

BodyGlide BodyGlide is a petroleum-free lubricant that protects against friction and skin irritation. This product comes in a "glide-on" applicator similar to a deodorant stick. BodyGlide is hypoallergenic, waterproof, non-sticky, non-greasy so it will not clog pores, and long lasting. Its main ingredients are triglycerides, aloe, and Vitamin E. Its applicator makes it awkward to use on toes but easy to apply to other areas. For more information contact BodyGlide, 11726 San Vicente Blvd, Suite 220, Los Angeles, CA 90049; (888) 263-9454; www.sternoff.com

Hydropel Hydropel Protective Silicone Ointment is an excellent foot lubricant. It is made with 30% silicone, petrolatum, dimethicone, and aluminum starch octonylsuccinate. It is also rated effective as a protectant against poison ivy. Offered in a two-ounce or one-pound size. Available only by mail order through C & M Pharmacal. C & M distributes the same product to medical specialists under the name Protective Barrier Ointment in their Essential Care product line. For more information contact C & M Pharmacal, 1721 Maplelane Avenue, Hazel Park, MI 48030; (800) 459-8663; www.hydropel.com

Lanolin Cream Some runners use lanolin cream on their feet. Lanolin hydrous is a natural topical skin emollient that lubricates, protects, and soothes. It usually comes in a small tube and may be found in most drug stores or pharmacies.

Runner's Lube Mueller makes Runner's Lube in a push-up tube. This anti-friction ointment contains lanolin, pain-relieving benzocaine, and zinc oxide. It can be found in sporting good stores. For more information contact Mueller Sports Medicine, Inc., One Quench Drive, Prairie du Sac, WI 53578; (800) 356-9522; www.muellersportsmed.com. Available through distributors or from Medco Sports Medicine (see page 273).

Skin-Lube　　Skin-Lube is a lubricating ointment that comes in a handy .55-ounce stick, a 2.75-ounce tube, or a one-pound jar. Its higher melting point gives it longer-lasting protection against blisters and chafing than petroleum jelly. Its main ingredients are petrolatum, zinc stearate, and silicone. Colorless and non-staining, it can be used on any friction-prone area of the body. It can be found in sporting good stores. For more information contact Cramer Products, Inc. PO Box 1001, Gardner, KS 66030; (800) 255-6621; www.cramersportsmed.com. Available through distributors or from Medco Sports Medicine (see page 273).

SportSlick　　Created by a sports physician, SportSlick is a multi-purpose lubricant made for athletes. The gel is easily applied to the toes, feet, inner thighs, underarms, nipples, and lips. SportSlick prevents blisters and chafing with antifriction polymers, silicone, and petrolatum which creates a silky feel. It also enriches the skin with Vitamin E and C, soybean oil, the antibacterial agent Triclosan, and the antifungal agent Tolnaftate 1%. SportSlick is available in one-ounce packets and a four-ounce tube. For more information contact SportSlick Products, 8930 Sepulveda Blvd, #206, Los Angeles, CA 90045; (800) 646-8448; www.sportslick.com.

Sportsloob　　Sportsloob is a cream that protects the skin against chafing. Its main ingredients are liquid paraffin, white petroleum jelly, and emulsifying wax. The odorless and colorless cream is activated by body heat and perspiration, providing a non-greasy shield for areas of the skin that make contact during motion. It is advertised as effective for 12 to 18 hours. For more information contact Sportsloob, PO Box 16693, Irvine, CA 92713-6693; (800) 525-LOOB.

Udder Balm　　Udder Balm has a lemon fragrance, is non-greasy, and is quickly absorbed by the skin. Similar to Bag Balm, Udder Balm was first made for cow udders, With ingredients including lanolin, aloe vera gel,, and vitamins A, D, and E, this cream is ideal for relief from rough, cracked skin, and also for corns, cracked cuticles, and sunburn. Udder Balm is available in four-ounce tubes, a one-pound jar, and a huge four-pound jar. For more information contact Udder Balm, 2953 Donita Drive, Birmingham, AL 35243; (205) 970-0622; www.cahaba.com/udderbalm.

Un-Petroleum Jelly   For those wanting a lubricant without petroleum, try Un-Petroleum Jelly. Made from natural plant oils and waxes, its ingredients are castor oil, coconut oil, PG-3 beeswax, sorbitan triteratre, silica, tocopherol (Vitamin E), and natural flavors. It soothes and moisturizes dry skin, prevents chafing and windburn, and is a general-purpose lubricant. Made by Autumn Harp, it is usually found in drug stores and health food stores. For more information contact Autumn Harp, 61 Pine Street, Bristol, Vermont 05443; (802) 453-4807.

Vaseline   Vaseline is available in three formulas. The old-time standard is 100% pure petroleum jelly. Newer formulas include Creamy Vaseline with Vitamin E and anti-bacterial Medicated Vaseline. The medicated formula, in particular, should be helpful for runner's feet, underarms, inner thighs, and nipples. Vaseline is available in most drug stores.

12

Skin Tougheners and Tape Adherents

Some athletes have found benefits against blisters by toughening the skin of their feet. Begin by spending time walking barefoot on various surfaces. Sandals, worn without socks, can build calluses, but be careful that the calluses do not become too thick or rough. As the skin is irritated, through exposure to rough surfaces, it thickens and calluses develop. Remember to keep calluses and roughened skin surfaces smooth by using creams, a pumice stone, or a foot file (see the chapters *Nutrition for the Feet* on page 121 and *Corns, Calluses, Bunions, and Bursitis* on page 241).

There are several products which can be used as skin tougheners or choose the tea and Betadine soak. Several of the products can also be used as tape adherents to help your choice of tape or moleskin better adhere to the feet. Let the spray dry completely before applying any tape. Be sure to apply a light coating of powder over any dried-sprayed area to counteract the adhesive. Without the adherent, most tapes and blister products will begin to peel off after an hour or two.

When using tincture of benzoin or a benzoin-based product, be sure to allow it time to dry. Generally three minutes' drying time is sufficient before applying any tape or blister product. Wet benzoin is very sticky and slippery. Tape and blister care products can move around on the foot and fold over on themselves creating problems. Socks can become glued to your feet and toes can stick together if you do not allow the benzoin time to dry.

Products

Cramer Tuf-Skin   Cramer's Tuf-Skin spray has been used for years by athletic trainers as a taping base. It is ideal for pre-taping and skin toughening. Its main ingredients are isopropyl alcohol, isobutane, resin, and benzoin. The original spray is available in an eight-ounce size while the colorless formula is available in four-, six-, and ten-ounce sizes. For more information contact Cramer Products, Inc. PO Box 1001, Gardner, KS 66030; (800) 255-6621; www.cramersportsmed.com. Available through distributors or from Medco Sports Medicine (see page 273).

Mueller Tuffner Clear Spray   This clear spray is used as a base for athletic taping, but is also identified as a skin toughener. Its main ingredients are acetone, 1,1,1-trichloroethanem isopropanol, resin, and tincture of benzoin. Look for this product at sporting good stores. For more information contact Mueller Sports Medicine, Inc., One Quench Drive, Prairie du Sac, WI 53578; (800) 356-9522; www.muellersportsmed.com. Available through distributors or from Medco Sports Medicine (see page 273).

New-Skin   New-Skin Liquid Bandage comes in either an antiseptic spray or liquid that is useful as a skin protectant or toughener to prevent hot spots and blisters. It dries rapidly to form a tough protective cover that is antiseptic, flexible, and waterproof, while letting the skin breathe. The one-ounce size is small and convenient. Clean the skin, spray or coat, and let dry. A second coating may be added for additional protection. Keep toes bent when applying and drying. There is no residue or stickiness. Do not apply to infected or draining sites. It is strong smelling stuff, so use with good ventilation and avoid breathing too deeply. Its main ingredients are pyroxylin solution, acetone ACS, oil of cloves, and 8-hydroxyquinoline. Look for New-Skin at drug stores. For more information contact Medtech Laboratories Inc. PO Box 1683, Jackson, WY 83001; (800) 443-4908.

Rubbing Alcohol   Renown walker Colin Fletcher suggests using rubbing alcohol on feet as a skin toughener.[14] Use it on your toes, soles, and heels several times daily. While walking and hiking with sore feet, he uses almost hourly applications of rubbing alcohol followed by foot powder. Rubbing alcohol is available in most drug stores.

Tuf-Foot   Tuf-Foot is made from nature's healing balsams and other ingredients:. This unique and original compound was made in 1935 by Dr. Andrew Bonn and has been used by veterinarians and trainers for over 60 years. Made exclusively for feet, either human and animal, Tuf-Foot is guaranteed to toughen soft, tender or sore feet by toughening the tissues. This protects against bruises, blisters, and foot soreness. Available in liquid form. Recommended use is daily until feet are in good condition and then twice weekly. For more information contact Bonaseptic Company, The Roberts Building-Suite 107, 2996 Grandview Avenue, NE, Atlanta, GA 30305; (888) 883-3668; www.tuffoot.com

Tincture of Benzoin   Tincture of benzoin is available in liquid, swabs, or squeeze vials. Commonly used as a tape or bandage adherent, it is sometimes used as a skin toughener. After applying the tincture, let it dry for about three minutes before applying tape. Tincture of benzoin leaves an orange-brownish color on the skin. Avoid getting the tincture into any cuts, abrasions, or open blisters—it can burn! Usually available in a liquid at drug stores, pharmacies, or medical supply stores. The swabs or squeeze vials may require a special order.

Tom Crawford's Tea and Betadine Skin Toughener
Tom Crawford is an ultrarunner who has completed numerous ultras including the challenging Death Valley to Mt. Whitney ultra both one way and as an out-and-back run. Tom's method begins with mixing ten Lipton tea bags and one cup of Betadine into ½-gallon of water. For one week, dip your feet 20 times over the course of a day, letting them air dry between dips. The second week, add one cup of salt to the water, tea, and Betadine mixture. Then for one week, soak your feet for 20 minutes at a time, several times daily. Betadine can be found in drug stores and medical supply stores.

Richard Benyo recalled how he used Tom's method to prepare his feet for the Death Valley 300. "Each night I'd pour the solution into a plastic foot bath and keep my soles and toes in the solution for fifteen minutes; then I'd alternately raise one foot out of the brew for three minutes, allowing it to dry, then lower it and bring the other foot out. I'd do that for a half-hour. Then I'd let them dry and I'd go to bed with orange soles. When I showered the next morning, it would wash off. But little by little, it made my feet more resistant to blisters."[15] Even with this preparation, Richard sometimes found his feet often susceptible to blisters.

13

Taping for Blisters

If your feet are prone to blistering, taping may be a lifesaver. After 12 hours of a 72-hour run, my Vaseline-coated feet were almost too sore to run on, and I had a blister between two toes. Nancy Crawford, an experienced running friend, taught me how to prepare my feet for taping and use duct tape to both fix the blister and tape the tender balls of my feet which would likely blister in the hours ahead. I completed the next 60 hours without a foot problem! While you may consider duct taping an extreme, consider the benefits of taping if you are highly susceptible to blisters. You can tape before your event as a proactive preventive measure or in a reactive mode after hot spots or blisters develop. Tape can be applied to more than feet. Rich Lewis finds that applying duct tape to his socks over where he typically develops hot spots or blisters, particularly in new shoes, is a good prevention measure. Other use duct tape inside their shoes or boots to cover irritating seams in their footwear.

Taping Basics

There are several types of tape available to try. Duct tape is the standard most often used. The Johnson & Johnson's Elastikon and 3M's Medipore and Microfoam tapes can be found at or ordered through most medical supply stores or from Medco Sports Medicine (see page 273).

- Duct tape is a 2″ wide, very sticky silver tape with a fabric core that has excellent adhesive qualities. Duct tape is available at any hardware store.
- Elastikon from Johnson & Johnson Medical Inc. is a medium-thickness elastic porous tape that comes in 1″, 2″, 3″, and 4″ widths.
- 3M's Medipore is a thin, soft knit-style tape which comes in 1″, 2″, 3″, and 4″ widths and is perforated in easy-to-tear strips. This tape conforms nicely to the contours of the feet.
- 3M's Microfoam is a 1/32″ thick, soft foam tape that comes in a 1″, 2″, and 4″ widths.

Runners who decide to try taping should purchase a tape adherent that provides a taping base to hold the tape to the skin. The best adherents are Cramer Products' Tuf-Skin spray, Mueller's Tuffner Clear Spray, or tincture of benzoin in a liquid or swabs. (See the chapter *Skin Tougheners and Tape Adherents* on page 87). These products help the tape adhere to the skin. Remember to let the tape adherent dry before applying the tape. After spraying and taping your feet, be sure to apply a sprinkling of powder to the sprayed areas that are not taped to counteract any adhesive left uncovered.

Preparation includes several steps. Before taping, clean the feet of their natural oils, dust, and dirt. Rubbing alcohol works well to clean the feet and dries quickly. For fanny pack use, buy alcohol wipes in small disposable packets. Next apply the tape adherent to the areas needing taping and let dry. Then apply the tape based on your specific needs or problems.

Keep the tape as smooth as possible. Ridges in the tape may cut into the skin and lead to irritation that may cause blisters. If the tape must be overlapped, be sure the overlapping edge of the tape is in the same direction as the force of motion. For example, if taping the ball of the foot, the force is towards the rear of the foot, so the most forward piece of tape should overlap over the piece towards the back. If taping the heel, the force is towards the rear and up the back of the heel, so the tape on the bottom of the heel should overlap the piece higher up on the back of the heel. This will keep the tape from catching on the sock and peeling up. The less overlap the better. Applying the tape too tight may cause circulation problems. If, after application, the skin becomes discolored, cool, or numb, loosen the tape.

Place a single layer of toilet paper or tissue over any existing blisters where the outer skin has pulled loose from the inner skin. This keeps the adhesive from attacking the sensitive area and protects the blistered skin when the tape is removed. You can also substitute a piece of duct tape for the tissue, sticky side to sticky side. This allows the slick side of the duct tape to face the hot spot or blister. Try not to use gauze since it is to abrasive.

After the foot is taped, several finishing touches should be made. Run a thin layer of Bag Balm, Vaseline or similar lubricant over the tape and around the edges. This reinforces the tape's status as part of your foot by providing a barrier that neutralizes any adhesive leaks and allows the taped surface to slip easily across friction points without snagging. Finally use a lubricant or powder on your feet to cut the sticky pre-tape base, if one was used.

You may be able to tape all areas of your feet yourself. If you have problems reaching the outer edges of your feet, your heels, or any other awkward area, find someone to help with the taping.

When removing the duct tape, work slowly and carefully. You would not want to pull off a layer of skin or a toenail with the tape. Work from the sides to the center, using the fingers of one hand to hold the skin while pulling the tape with the other hand. Ultrarunner Suzi Cope suggests using baby oil and gentle massage to roll off the tape and excessive adhesive.

Taping is useful for pre-run preparation as well as to fix newly developed problem spots. If you typically blister on the balls of your feet, consider taping before the run when you have the time to do it right rather then at an aid station when you need every minute of time. Practice taping to learn how best to apply the tape to meet your particular needs. Determine how much time is needed to do a complete application. If you are going to have crew support for an event, teach them how to do the taping. It is usually easier to tape the night before an event than wait until the morning when time is rushed and you may do a hurried job.

Below are two methods of taping the feet. The first uses duct tape. The second uses Johnson & Johnson Elastikon tape. Each method can be used with the other types of tape mentioned earlier. If you are bothered by blisters, and have found that powders and/ or lubricants do not work, try the different tapes to find a tape and taping method, which works for you. In the chapter *Foot Care Kits* on page 261 you will find a list of taping materials to carry during your runs and hikes.

Duct Tape Techniques

Duct tape is tough. In 1968, *Popular Mechanics*, in their New Products column, reviewed Arno Adhesive's "duct tape." They casually noted it was also ideal for "... other jobs around the house." Little did they know that the silver duct tape would become a staple in the athlete's footcare kit. A mail order catalog offers a T-shirt with a picture of the familiar silver roll and the words "When the Going Gets Tough, The Tough Use Duct Tape." Ultrarunner Ivy Franklin blistered so badly at the Arkansas Traveller 100 in 1994 that she dropped at 68 miles. Then she learned about the miracle of duct taping and ran the Umstead Trail 100 in 1995 and returned to the Arkansas Traveller 100 in 1996 without either blisters or hot spots.

Many runners have successfully used Gary Cantrell's article "From the South: The Amazing Miracle of Duct Tape"[16] to learn how to prevent and treat blisters. Gary's basic principle is to cover the spot that's injured with a patch and in some cases then anchor the edges and corners of that patch. The powerful adhesive of duct tape holds it true to the outline of your skin and the tough, plastic outer tape skin reinforced with fabric can withstand almost unlimited friction. The friction points on your skin will then have an additional layer of skin—the duct tape. Gary's method follows, with a few of my time-tested additions.

Remember a few general duct tape rules. Choose a good quality duct tape with a visible fabric core, not a plastic cheap imitation. Many hardware stores carry several types of duct tape. The standard grade is typically nine-mil thick while the contractor and professional grades are generally ten-mil thick. Duct tape is only available in a 2″ width. Although the tape is sometimes available in a variety of colors the common silver tape works the best.

The tape is applied over the danger spots where blisters frequently occur. Don't apply tape where it is not needed. Use only a single thickness since additional layers become too hard and unyielding. When the tape is applied, that part of the foot should be flexed to its maximum extension. Cut the ends of the tape so they are rounded. If your feet are hairy, shave the parts where the tape will be applied.

Generally speaking, with duct tape do not tape all the way around toes or the foot because of possible circulation problems. If after applying tape, the skin or portion of the foot farthest from the body becomes discolored, cool, or numb, loosen the tape.

Taping the ball of the foot   Take a long strip of full-width tape and place it, adhesive side up, on the floor. Place your foot on it at a right angle, with the trouble spot dead center on the tape. Then flatten your foot to make it as wide as possible and pull the ends of the tape up, either overlapping them on the top of your foot or cutting them an inch up on either side of the foot. Cut the tape at the forward edge of the ball of the foot so it does not contact or cut into the crease at the base of the toes or the toes themselves.

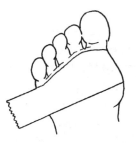

Cut tape to conform to the
shape of the forefoot

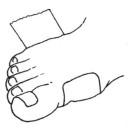

Wrap tape up the sides
of the foot

Taping the toes   First tear off a small strip and use
it to wrap from the base of the toenail around the tip of the toe and
to the bottom of the toe even with the end on top, leaving two free
ends. (Omit this step for toes that don't blister at the tip.) Wrap
another strip around the circumference of the toe, covering the
free ends of the first strip, if it was used. Have the two end meet
but try to avoid overlap them on top of the toe. Always use a large
enough strip to cover the toe's "knuckle joint" so that both outside
edges are too small to slide over the joint and cause the tape to
bunch off or slip off the end of the toe. Never extend the edge far
enough down that it will dig into the tender skin between the toes.
For taping against toenail friction, tape the receiving toe, rather
than the offending nail.

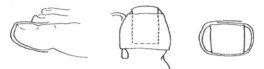

Use two pieces of tape for toes, one from top to
bottom over the tip and another around the toe

Taping between toe and foot   Cut a small pad of sterile gauze or tissue and place it firmly over the blister. Fasten it in
place with a slightly larger square of tape. Take a long thin strip of
tape and run it diagonally, corner to corner, between your toes
from the top of your foot to the ball of your foot. Take another
long, thin strip and do the same with the two remaining corners.
Now you have a pad on the blister, the pad protected by duct tape,
and the whole thing held firmly in place by the four strips attaching the corners to the tops and bottoms of your feet. Now anchor
these strips with the single piece described for the ball of the foot,
and the most difficult blister of all is fixed.

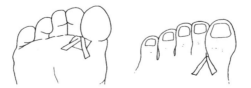

Two diagonal strips of tape anchors the patch over a blister

Taping the bottom of the heel   Remember when applying duct tape to the bottoms of your feet or heels grasp the toes of the foot and pull back to stretch the skin to its fullest. Otherwise as you run or walk there will be shear forces that will loosen the tape and may cause additional blisters. Start with a large patch of tape covering the entire heel. Attach it with both the foot and ankle flexed forward and up (pull your toes toward your shin). Take a long strip of tape cut to a 1″ width and cover the forward edge of the patch under your foot and bring the ends up to overlap on top of the foot. Take another medium strip and cover the edge on the back of your heel and bring the ends around the ankle to overlap on top of the first strip.

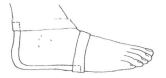

Tape under the foot, up the heel, and secure it with two strips around the foot

Suzi's Taping Techniques

Suzi Cope, an ultrarunner, developed this taping technique while completing the Grand Slam of trail ultrarunning, five 100-mile runs in one summer with only a couple of small "tape" blisters. Suzi stresses this technique will not work for everybody. Your individual footprint and running style may affect the taping. Suzi's technique involves taping the bottom of each foot up to the heel, around the sides of the foot, and each toe. She recommends taping the night before an event after taking a shower. She has often had the tape on up to 36 hours without a problem.

Suzi uses Johnson & Johnson's Elastikon tape in 2″ and 4″ widths. River and stream crossings are not a problem since the tape is porous and dries as fast as socks and shoes. Do not stretch the tape, simply form it to the foot and press firmly. All points where the tape folds or is pinched together should be folded like a gift-wrap fold and cut flush with the skin. This is truly preventative maintenance, creating a sock type effect. Determine your specific hot spot or blister problems and try taping as needed. When cutting the tape flush with the skin, be careful not to cut the skin. She recommends baby oil and gentle massage to remove the tape.

Suzi technique uses the following three steps to tape the whole foot. If you only have problems on the ball of the foot, the heels, or the toes, use the appropriate taping strategy.

Taping the bottom of the foot   Apply a 4″ piece of tape from just behind the bend of the toe base, centering the tape on the bottom of the foot from front to back. Have equal edges on the inside and outside of the foot. Trim the front edge to follow the contour of the toe base avoiding the crease. Bring the back edge up the heel and fold over on each side, like a gift- wrap, making a dart. Cut the fold flush with the foot, leaving two edges just meeting in a "V" pattern.

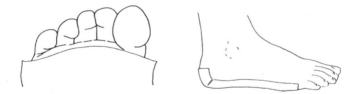

Center the tape on the foot to allow equal amounts up the sides of the foot, cut to the shape of the forefoot, and mold up the heel

Taping the sides of the foot   Once the 4″ piece is in place on the bottom of the foot, apply a 2″ piece around the foot from one side to the other. Slightly overlap over the edge of the 4″ tape. Trim the edges to avoid rubbing at the toe crease and ankle-bone. If you find the bottom edge of the tape catching on your socks, put this layer on before taping the bottom of the foot. Then tape the bottom of the foot so that tape overlaps the side of the foot tape. This method keeps the overlapping tape in the direction of the force of motion as described earlier.

Apply a single strip of tape around the back of the heel, overlapping the bottom of the foot piece

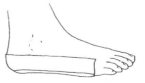

Taping the toes Toes are taped with pieces of the 2″ tape. Tape only the last two joints, avoiding the crease at the base of the toes. Roll the tape around the toe, over-lapping over the toenails for a double-layer but keeping a single-layer on the sides of the toes. Fold the excess over at the tips of the toes, pinching the top and bottom together. Cut the tape flush with the skin, leaving no overlap. Since Elastikon tape is stretchy, the overlapping of the tape is not an issue here as it is with duct tape.

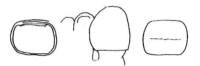

Tape toes with one piece around the toe, pinch it
closed and cut it flush with the skin

14

151 Ways to Prevent Blisters

Most athletes hold a common misconception about blisters—that blisters are simply a fact of life that one must learn to live with. Most athletes try tips that they have learned from others. If those don't work, they move on to another idea. Most try for a while, then give up and spend the rest of their life fixing their inevitable blisters. The fact is, there are many ways to prevent blisters.

Adventure racer Dan O'Shea has spent eight years learning what works for him in preventing blisters, "I have trained my feet for the stress of my sport and they have a tough outer layer. For races, I use tincture of benzoin, followed by Sports Slick lubricant, and then a double-sock system." At the 1999 Beast of the East Adventure Race he raced with two first-timers whose feet were hardly conditioned to the rigors of a five-day race. After two days of racing Dan found that, "Both these individuals had blisters on top of blisters and could walk only with great pain." Dan and teammate Harald Zundel, both former Navy SEALs and experienced racers, had maybe one blister between the two of them. His story is a good example of how important it is to find what works for *your feet*. Over the years he has learned different blister prevention techniques that work best on his feet. But he also realizes that what works for him may change over time as he gets new or different shoes, as his feet change, and as he participates in different types of events under changing conditions. Dan has the right approach—keep on learning and always be open to new blister prevention ideas.

Understand that while the blister prevention techniques you currently use may work today, they may not work tomorrow. Knowing what options are available will help you be prepared. The ideas that follow show the improvising spirit of athletes. Try one or two, then try a few more to find the ones that work for you.

Things You Do To Your Feet

Many athletes believe they that what they do to their feet helps prevent blisters. They have identified many options that are worth trying.

1. Toughen the skin on your feet by walking and running barefoot on grass, dirt, and sand. —Matt Mahoney
2. I pamper my feet with a pedicure. —Veronica Williams
3. I keep my feet as soft as a baby's bottom. —Dave Scott
4. Form calluses on your feet.
5. Keep your toenails clipped short. —Pat & Walt Radney
6. I don't get blisters when my feet are wet! I even did my feet in streams. —Lisa Demoney
7. Keep your feet dry by changing socks whenever possible. — Mike Snow
8. Lightly sandpaper your feet every few days. —Mike Snow
9. For a week before I pack or race, I soak the soles of my feet in rubbing alcohol. —George Cole
10. Three days before an event, I apply an antiperspirant (Ban Roll-on) to all skin surfaces up to the ankles, especially between the toes. —George Cole
11. The more you run the tougher your feet will get. —Mike Snow
12. Give yourself foot massages whenever you can. —Karen Borski
13. Blisters and most other foot problems can be avoided altogether by hiking in bare feet.
14. Use a callus cream to soften calluses and prevent friction and resulting blisters.

15. One way to prevent blisters sounds strange but works. Boil oak or hickory bark or twigs in water 5-15 minutes. Allow the water to cool. This makes a mild solution of tannic acid. Soaking feet in this solution will "tan" the skin on your feet and will help prevent blisters. —Carl Schmid
16. My feet may have been in better shape from the running, but they weren't tough enough to deal with the stress that a pack was causing. You must train your feet also. —Brick Robbins
17. I don't get blisters when my feet are wet.
18. Keep your feet soft and supple. I get a pedicure at least once a month smoothing out all calluses and rough spots, and put creams on my feet on a daily basis. When I hit the trails or roads, I use foot powder. Things have improved greatly. — Dave Littlehales

Things You Apply to Your Feet

There are many things you can apply to your feet to help prevent blisters. Lubricants and tape are two of the most popular. Powders are a distant third. Remember that whatever you apply to your feet will react to what you put around your feet. When you apply a lubricant, your socks will pickup some of it, and more applications will be necessary. Tape works well, but tape applied poorly can be pulled loose as you pull on your socks.

19. Use Bag Balm as a lubricate to reduce friction. —Robert Blackwell
20. Apply Vaseline to your feet. —Annie, Phil Mislinski and Bob Slate
21. Johnson & Johnson Elastikon tape is great preventative medicine! It is porous and easier on your skin than duct tape. — Suzi Cope and Pat Wellington
22. Use strapping tape.
23. Apply five-inch strips of "cloth" style duct tape on the heels, the bottom front of the foot, and the toes. —John H

24. Apply Johnson & Johnson athletic tape over the spots that have a been a problem in the past. —Karl King
25. Coat your feet with Hydropel Silicone Protective Ointment.
26. Duct tape known hot spots or problem areas. —George Cole, Bret Edge and Jeffrey Olson
27. Use Sports Slick lubricant each time you change your socks. —Dan O'Shea
28. Use Tincture of benzoin to bond Blister Relief pad to your problem spots. —Jeff Wold
29. Use Spenco 2nd Skin covered with moleskin. —Rob Langsdorf
30. Rub your feet with rubbing alcohol every day for a month before starting a long hike.
31. Apply New-Skin Liquid Bandage in several layers over hot spots. —Kojac and Plodder
32. Use Gold Bond Powder, it is a an indispensable cure-all for blisters.
33. Apply lanolin to your feet.
34. Apply Udder Balm as a lubricant.
35. Used clear nail polish in layers over hot spots. —Kojac
36. Use Avon's Silcone Glove cream to reduce friction.
37. Apply Tuf-Foot to toughen and protect your feet.
38. Use Zeasorb super absorbent powder on your feet.
39. Spray Mueller's Tuffner Clear Spray on your feet to toughen your skin.
40. Use Andrew Lovy's formula of A and D Ointment, Vaseline, Desitin ointment, vitamin E cream, and Aloe Vera cream.
41. Put moleskin over hot spots.
42. Duct tape really does fix everything. Placed over second skin, or other sterile bandaging, it prevent wear on the skin. —Sandra Kemper
43. Apply Band-Aid Blister Relief strips around your toes to prevent toe blisters. —Scott Weber
44. Use foot powder at every opportunity. —Karen Borski
45. Use adhesive felt, it is thicker than moleskin and sticks better.
46. Wash your feet every night when out on a hiking trip. —Karen Borski
47. We plastered our feet in a substance called Sudocrem twice a

day during a big race. Primarily designed to prevent diaper rash, this antiseptic healing cream leaves an oily trace on your feet and lasts for ages. —Brian Elliot

48. Use BodyGlide lubricant.
49. I put Band-Aid Blister Relief on any blister-prone spots prior to any race.
50. Apply multiple coats of tincture of benzoin to your feet as a toughener.

Things You Put Around Your Feet

What you put around your feet is one of the most important factors in blister prevention. The wrong type of socks, shoes or boots that fit wrong creating pressure points, and modifying your footwear can all help. This is an area where trying different ideas can really pay off.

51. Use two socks, a thin liner sock made of silk or polypropylene, with your favorite outer sock on top. —Dan O'Shea
52. Wear two pair of thin socks. —Buzz Burrell
53. Avoid cotton socks, they retain moisture.
54. Wear socks with Blister-Guard's Teflon Fibers.
55. Duct tape your socks in areas where you tend to blister. — Rick Lewis
56. I've had good luck putting pieces of lamb's wool coated with lanolin between the toes. This soft fibrous padding is usually available in the foot section of most drug stores and pharmacies. The natural lanolin in the wool was a break through, because no matter how well or completely I tape my toes, I blistered between them. —Ray Zirblis
57. To prevent heel blisters, put a piece of lambswool in the heel of the sock. —Joanne Lennox
58. Don't wear polypropylene sock liners. Until I threw mine away, I had horrible blisters which I had to duct tape. —BettySue Allen

59. Be sure to smooth the heels of your socks, and check the heels of your insoles and the inside of your heel counters for folds and worn or torn material. —Jay Hodde
60. Well cushioned shoes. —Veronica Williams
61. Duct tape rough areas inside your boots.
62. Once I find a pair of shoes that fits well and works for my running style and choice of terrain I buy at least six pair. — Phil Mislinski
63. To prevent heel blisters at the bottom back edge of the heel, where the insole meets the foot, put a small piece of lambswool or sheepskin on the edge of the insole to fill that space. — Joanne Lennox
64. Take time to really test a new boot before leaving the store. I usually wear mine around the store for an hour or more before deciding to take it. It takes time, but consumes less time than having to return it or having to spend lots of time treating blisters. —Rob Langsdorf
65. Use sheepskin and lambswool. In a pinch you can cut the top off ragg socks or by unraveling the sock and getting a bunch of yarn just use the whole wad. —Joanne Lennox
66. Break in new boots in by wearing them around the house, to work, church, etc. before going out on the trail. Then begin with some easy hikes before starting off on a long trip. Only when they feel good on a short hike are they ready for a longer one. —Rob Langsdorf
67. If you haven't worn your old boots for sometime, always take at least one break in walk in them before going on a major hike. Your foot may have changed and it may need to get reacquainted with the boot before making a long hike with it. — Rob Langsdorf
68. Switch from leather boots to running shoes for hiking and modify them with your knife if they feel too tight or hurt. — Kojac
69. Always wear SmartWool ultra thin running socks, they are great at wicking, dry quickly, and cause no irritation. —Phil Mislinski.
70. Replace worn out shoes. —Kojac

71. Get boots that fit properly. —Cynthia Taylor-Miller
72. To keep your feet dry, look for shoes and boots with good ventilation. —Cynthia Taylor-Miller
73. Wear socks inside out. The seam that goes across the toes can rub the tops and sides of the toes and cause blisters. —Cynthia Taylor-Miller
74. Wear liner socks.
75. Wear SealSkinZ waterproof socks.
76. Well made orthotics will help prevent blisters.
77. Weave strips of lambs wool between your toes and around the tips of your toes, and add more as needed. Wash it occasionally to restore its loft and cushioning. —Michael Henderson
78. The heel is the first part of the sock to wear thin, get new socks before they get too threadbare. —Kevin Corcoran
79. Unless it's quite cold I wear well-ventilated trail running shoes when on the trail. —George Cole
80. Use shoes that are tested for the event and the distance. Have one model for cold-weather and another for trails in warm and/or wet conditions. —Doug McKeever
81. Wear Gore-tex fabric socks.
82. Wear three pairs of socks, the first pair is a wicking sock, then regular socks. —Matthew Jankowicz
83. Wear rock climber's socks. They are thin and fit snugly. — Will Uher
84. To drain out sweat and water, use a red hot nail to burn drain holes on the sides of your shoes right at the sock liner height where the shoe bends. —Jim Stroup
85. Check a new pair of shoes or boots for problem areas, even if they are the same brand and size as your last pair. —Joanne Lennox
86. Coolmax socks do an excellent job of wicking moisture away from the feet. —Paul Alsop
87. Wear shoe gaiters to keep rocks, dust, and dirt out of the shoes, which means that the socks stay cleaner longer. —Paul Alsop
88. Once I switched to another pair of shoes the blisters went away. Many shoes breathe better than others and are better on your feet.

89. For hiking I use an old pair of combat boots with the toes cut off about three inches across the top of the toes. Have a shoe shop sew a strip of leather about one-inch wide across the boot to re-enforce the opening. This makes all five toes visible on both feet and saves the toes. —Billie M Thrash

90. First duct tape all problem areas, then apply a light coating of lubricant to your feet, put the first sock on each foot, apply more lubricant to the foot section of the socks, and then put on the second pair of socks. —Dalton Pulsipher Jr.

91. Put a patch of lamb's wool on a bruised, sore, or blistered area and secure it to the foot with duct tape. —Scott Weber

Things You Do in Combinations

Some blister prevention ideas work best in combination with other ideas. Vaseline and wicking socks. Tincture of benzoin to hold tape on the feet. Skin tougheners and double-layer socks. The list goes on and on, everything from using an antiperspirant to using motor oil!

92. Vaseline your feet, then pull on ankle length nylons, followed by socks and then shoes. —Geraldine Wales

93. Use Ultimax socks and a thin coat of Vaseline. —Jim Stroup

94. Apply Medicated A and D Ointment to your feet the night before a race, then the socks you will run in the next day. Reapply the ointment in the morning and use the same socks. —Scott Snyder

95. Wear shoes that fit a little big and double-layer socks, and stay well-hydrated. —Jay Hodde

96. Apply tincture of benzoin to the bottom and sides of the foot. Then with the foot in a relaxed position, layer strips of athletic tape from the back of the heel to the front of the foot, with each piece slightly overlapping the previous piece. — Chalres Steele

97. Try to keep your feet dry, air them out at breaks, and change

from wet socks to dry ones. —Cynthia Taylor-Miller

98. Spray your feet with Cramer's Tuf Skin, followed by Hydropel Silicone Protective Ointment. —Dr. Billy Tolan

99. Use a combination of thin Coolmax socks, frequent sock changes, re-lubricating with bag balm every 25 miles, and continous fluid and salt intake. —Bill Ramsey.

100. Spray your feet with New-Skin Liquid Bandage, wear nylon hose, then double-layer socks, all this inside of extra-long and extra-wide shoes. —Nikki Robinson

101. Use Tom Crawford's Lipton Tea and Betadine soak as a skin toughener.

102. Spray the soles of your feet with Cramer's Tuf-Skin or an equivalent. Two coats is better, allowing the first to dry a minute. Let it dry a minute or so until tacky, then roll on a pair of the two-layer cool max double-layer socks. The tacky spray causes the inner layer of the two-layer sock to bond to your foot. All the slippage, and friction, thus occurs between the two layers of the sock, or between the sock and the shoe. — Pierre Redmond

103. Clean your feet thoroughly. Coat your heels, toes, and soles with tincture of benzoin. After it dries, apply a layer of Avon Silicone Glove, followed by double-layer socks. Reapply every four to six hours and change socks at the same time. — Marvin Skagerberg

104. Wear good shoes and socks that fit properly. —Dennis Halpin

105. Wear Duraspun acrylic socks with lots of foot powder.

106. Use duct tape, foot powder, and synthetic socks. —David Burroughs

107. I use antiperspirant (Ban Roll-on) every morning of the event before I put on my socks. —George Cole

108. Wear Coolmax socks, with duct tape on the sock over the areas where the hot spots are or will be, and a second pair of socks over this combination. You must remove the duct tape from the sock and soak the sock in hot soapy water as soon as possible to remove the duct tape glue. —Rick

109. I pre-tape my feet in areas where I know from past experi-

ence I have had blisters and use shoes that on non-taped feet have not caused blisters on shorter runs. It isn't taping or the shoes, it's both. —Doug McKeever

110.   Shave the hair off your feet and duct-tape them before you leave the house.

111.   I recommend new motor oil, basic cheap oil works great. No special weight, but I try to stay away from oils with additives. Then cheap men's 50/50 cotton polyester socks from any discount department store. The 100% synthetic seem to work also, but I'm too cheap to buy them. Remember though, the oil must be new since used oil is a carcinogenic. —Ray Krolewicz

112.   The night before a run apply Cramer Tuf-Skin. In the morning rub on Vaseline and coat with baby powder, followed by nylon socks, more powder, and then thick socks. —Scott Rafferty

113.   Use two Coolmax socks that allow motion between the two layers and not with the feet. —Paul Alsop

114.   Wear nylons under wool socks (for hiking). —Mary Gorski

115.   Dry feet and good clean socks are the best prevention for blisters.

116.   I first spray the bottom, sides and blister prone parts of my feet with tincture of benzoin and let it dry. At first I use to cut strips of duct tape but now use 3M Microfoam tape. Stretch it slightly as you put it on and smooth out any bumps. —G. Velasco

117.   I use women's nylon ankle stockings on my feet first, followed by a double- or single-layer Coolmax socks. —Ray Zirblis

118.   I wear a Coolmax liner sock with either Thorlo Coolmax blend light hiking socks (summer) or Smartwool hiking socks (winter). —George Cole

119.   I learned to wash my feet as seldom as possible and wear the same socks most of the time. My feet developed a protective layer of dead skin and dirt that made them nearly bulletproof. Blisters and abrasions never developed. —Andrew Perdas

120.   Change the liner and sock for a second pair about once every two hours (or less if it's really warm) and let the original pair dry out. —George Cole

121.   Wash off your feet at night and coat with Vaseline. —Walt & Pat

Things You Do in General

In addition to doing things to your feet, applying things to your feet, being careful to what you put around your feet, there are other ideas that are helpful in preventing blisters. The ideas here run the gamut from lacing techniques, hydration, proper shoe and boot fit, and regular changes of socks.

122.   Drink a lot of water to stay hydrated. —John H

123.   Stay properly hydrated with electrolytes to maintain good sodium levels. —Karl King

124.   Learn different lacing techniques to prevent your feet from slipping inside the shoes.

125.   The key is prevention, think of boot, socks, epidermis, and lower skin layers as a "system" and to treat the whole system. —Tom McGinnis

126.   Some insoles are better than others at helping to prevent blisters.

127.   Re-lace your shoelaces in a different lace configuration to take the pressure off a hot spot. —Pat & Walt Radney

128.   Above all else, make sure the shoes fit. —Buzz Burrell

129.   Wear new boots around the house to break them in before hitting the trail.

130.   Elevate your feet during breaks and at night to keep swelling down.

131.   Run without socks to keep your feet from sliding around in your shoes and get a better grip on the soles of your shoes. —Matt Mahoney

132.   Two months before a race do lots of running sessions with

bare feet on sand. —Mike Snow

133. Stop and check out "hot spots" before they turn into blisters. —Rob Langsdorf

134. Slow down if you feet start to over heat. Often this allows the feet to cool enough to keep from blistering. —Rob Langsdorf

135. Rotate between several pairs of shoes. —Jon Drury

136. Use Superfeet insoles. —Walt & Pat

137. For extreme heat, I cut up a space blanket on all the non-white parts of my shoes and under the insole. —Clive Saffery

138. I wore boots that were slightly too large so that during the course of a hike, as my feet naturally swelled, they wouldn't become too tight and rub.

139. I started hiking with a pack on every weekend. After initial blisters, calluses finally developed which helped toughen my feet.

140. Don't sleep in damp socks. —Karen Borski

141. Change your socks regularly.

142. Don't hike ultra-long days in wet boots. —Karen Borski

143. Wet feet are less a problem than is the dust, dirt, and tiny pebbles that work their way through your shoes. The mesh upper allows the grit in, and the sweat from your feet turns it to a mucky ooze that just invites trouble. Take a break at the aid stations and remove your shoes and socks, wipe your feet, pound out the dirt in the socks, and put everything back on. — Jay Hodde

144. If you are hiking in wet boots and socks, slow your pace a bit to reduce pressure on the skin of your feet. —Karen Borski

145. Allow your feet dry out as often as possible, including taking shoes-off breaks when out for a long hike. —Karen Borski

146. If blisters persist, get new shoes. —Karen Borski

147. Take your boots and socks off once an hour, religiously, to air your feet. —Jeffrey Olson

148. I trace the outline of my feet on an 8x11 paper after doing a 100-miler and sketch in the blisters, noting any anti-blister techniques I used. This helps me remember what I've tried

and what worked or didn't. —Ray Zirblis

149.   The guy at the outfitters who help me fit my boots correctly saved my feet.

150.   The best way I've found to prevent blisters is to get blisters. I don't do anything to avoid blisters on training runs and actually welcome it when I do get a blister because I know my feet are getting tougher. On race day it's different, then I go for the double socks, gaiters, comfortable shoes, etc. —Scott Diamond

And finally, ending on a humorous note, one more way to prevent blisters.

151.   I have discovered a 100% foolproof way of avoiding blisters. Its beauty lies in its simplicity, its effectiveness is unparalleled by any remedy to which I've been exposed, and it works just as well in the marathon/ultra-marathon world as it does in adventure racing. Here it is: at the start of the race, as everyone takes off, you elevate both feet (on a log, an ottoman, a slavish support crew member, or whatever) and if you can stay there until the race is over, blisters are guaranteed not to get you. —David Schmitt

15

Orthotics

Many runners wear an orthotic device in one or both shoes to help maintain the foot in a functionally correct position. Gait irregularities can be corrected. Support can be provided for flatfeet and pronation problems. Malalignment problems such as leg length inequality can be corrected. They can also relieve pressure by providing support behind a problem area as in a callous, neuroma, or metatarsal injury. Typically prescribed by a podiatrist or orthopedist, orthotics are medical devices made from cast impressions of your feet. A properly fit orthotic will control arch and pressure point problems.

The need for orthotics may begin with pain in your feet, repeated blistering in the same place on your feet from pressure, or even problems in your knees or hips as your gait is changed due to biomechanical stresses. Doug Mitchell tells, "I had substantial pain in the ball/metatarsal area many years ago. I was doing about 60 miles/week, and heavy lifting too, including very heavy calf raises. I turned out I had a minor structural problem in the foot which created a lot of stress on the ball of my feet. After a while, I went to see a podiatrist, resulting in my first orthotics which solved the problem." Doug uses his orthotics almost exclusively in his running and athletic footwear. Check with your health care plan to determine if they cover orthotics.

Custom-Made Orthotics

Custom-made orthotics may be soft, semi-rigid, or rigid, and are made specifically for your feet. They may be made in the pedorthists, podiatrists, or orthopedists office from common materials or custom made of special materials. Materials may include felt pads, cork, foam, viscoelastic, silicon, closed-cell rubber or closed-cell polyethylene, fiberglass, or leather. Orthotics can be made in various lengths and include metatarsal pads or heel wedges. They are made to work in partnership with your boots and shoes. Poor-quality boots and shoes may alter the corrective action of an orthotic.

In the article "The Ideal Running Orthosis: A Philosophy of Design,"[17] the authors build a case for the ideal orthotic. They recommend a custom fit in either semirigid or semiflexible design, lightweight, yet inexpensive, with a covering to decrease shear while giving control to both the forefoot and hindfoot, all while retaining memory in its shape and being adjustable at a later time. It also needs to be transferable to most of the client's shoes. They place orthotics in two categories of design: corrective and accommodative. A corrective orthotic should attempt, with a rigid design, to correct the foot's position so that its abnormal anatomy will mold to the corrected position. An accommodative orthotic should attempt to relieve areas of high stress or reposition the foot to better deal with its stress, usually with a soft or semiflexible design. The most common type of orthotic is semiflexible.

Your pedorthist, podiatrist, or orthopedist can ask the right questions and order the right tests to make the correct diagnosis of which type of corrective orthotic is necessary. The typical process includes a detailed injury history, complete lower-extremity biomechanical examination including a gait analysis, and a check of your shoes or boots. The aim is to identify the cause of your injury and try to prevent its continuation or recurrence. Orthotics may be prescribed for the treatment of plantar fasciitis, tendinitis, runner's knee, shin splints, lower back pain, and other conditions. Patient compliance in wearing the orthotic is the dominant issue in resolving foot problems. Modifications to the orthotics may be necessary to ensure a proper fit. If the orthotic is uncomfortable it will not be worn. Your should receive complete instructions on the use and care of your orthotics. Once using orthotics, and pain free, continue to use the orthotic as long as they work for your feet. Some injuries that require orthotics will be relieved after a short period of time, other gait and support, and foot function problems will require long-term use.

Ask your pedorthist, podiatrist, or orthopedist about what you need to do to help the orthotics work. He or she may give you a detailed treatment schedule of stretching and strengthening exercises and advice on shoe or boot selection. You may also be advised to wear the orthotics for several hours a day and gradually work your way up to longer periods.

If your foot seems to slip on your orthotic, ask about changing the surface material. A thin layer of Spenco insole material or your favorite insole material can usually be glued to the orthotic using rubber cement. The use of Spenco's Slip-In Insoles can add needed cushioning to your orthotics. These Slip-In Insoles can even be doubled up for added cushioning. TacTape can be used on an orthotic to prevent slipage.

Mail order orthotics need to be checked out thoroughly and purchased only through reputable companies. Adjustments to mail order orthotics can be difficult. Avoid drug store orthotics. Arch supports sold in sporting goods and drug stores should not be mistaken for orthotics. The Hapad, Lynco, and Spenco orthotics identified below are just three of many low cost orthotics that can be helpful as an alternative to custom orthotics and "quick-fix" drug store remedies.

Custom Orthotic Alternatives

There are alternatives to custom orthotics. Not everyone needs a custom orthotic and it may be worth your while to try one of two over-the-counter insoles. They may work. Some of these insoles are designed for specific foot problems

Nick Williams had "... tried hard orthotics, soft orthotics, Spenco orthotics, and just about anything else to keep my feet from hurting." Then an orthopedic surgeon told him about Hapads and gave him a pair. They have kept him pain free for the last five years and are flexible on trails. Nick now swears by Hapads and via e-mail told Ed Furtaw about them. Ed wore custom made orthotics for 10 years but now uses the Comf-Orthotic 3/4-length insoles, without heel pain, saying, "They are definitely more comfortable than wearing orthotics." Ed added the Hapad Scaphoid Pads for extra arch support. Now Ed's wife has switched from custom orthotics to the Comf-Orthotic. After an area on one arch got a little sore, they peeled away some of the wool material to make it fit better. Ed believes that "With something like Hapads, a person can take more responsibility for their own orthotic adjustments, which would be very difficult or impossible with custom-molded rigid orthotics." An orthopedist told me that if he had only one product to offer his patients, he would choose Hapads!

Products

Custom-made Orthotics   There are many custom made orthotics available and your pedorthist, podiatrist, or orthopedist will help select the correct one for your feet. The line of custom made orthotics and insoles is constantly changing.

- **MetaPumper Orthotics** – A custom fluid orthotic that changes its shape and characteristics as the foot goes through its heel strike to toe-off. Then fluid moves through the foot's motion, cushioning as it moves. Mark Medical, 1168-C Aster Avenue, Sunnyvale, CA 94086; (800) 433-FOOT.
- **Arch Crafters Custom-Fit Insoles**   These insoles are an example of what some stores offer to the general public. They are often used as a substitute for orthotics. AmFit uses a scanned image of your feet to make a custom insole. To find a store near you that uses this technology, contact AmFit Inc., 2850 Bowers Avenue, Santa Clara, CA 95951; (408) 986-1232; www.amfit.com.

Custom Insole Alternatives   The insoles listed below are proven alternatives to the more costly custom orthotics. Your podiatrist or pedorthist might be able to help find other models.

- **Hapad Comf-Orthotic** Hapad makes several orthotics that are popular because of their low cost and effectiveness. The 3/4-length and full-length insoles are helpful for heel spur pain and flat feet. The 3-Way Heel/Arch/Metatarsal Insole is a combination longitudinal metatarsal arch pad with a heel extension and is effective for plantar fasciitis. These three are made from coiled, spring-like wool fibers that provide firm and resilient support as they mold and shape to the foot. The full-length contoured Comf-Orthotic Sports Replacement Insole is made in three layers with a moisture-wicking suede top, a ventilated Poron middle layer for shock absorption, and a bottom of Microcel "Puff," a self-molding foot bed. The insole includes a metatarsal bar to relieve pressure at the ball of the foot, a medial arch support to limit pronation, and a heel cup for stability and control of the foot and ankle. For more information contact Hapad Inc., PO Box 6, 5301 Enterprise Blvd., Bethel Park, PA 15102; (800) 544-2723; www.hapad.com.
- **Lynco Biomechanical Orthotic Systems** Apex offers the Lynco Biomechanical Orthotic System, a "ready-made" triple-density orthotic system that comes in enough variations to accommodate 90% of foot disorders. By identifying your foot type as either normal, high arched, or flat/over pronated, a model is determined. Three basic models are offered: 1) heel pain related to heel spurs, heel pain syndrome, Achilles tendinitis, and plantar fasciitis; 2) arch pain related to arch strain, post-tib tendinitis, and plantar fasciitis; and 3) metatarsal pain related to metatarsalgia, Morton's toe, and Morton's neuroma. Each model, based on foot type, comes with either a neutral-cupped heel or a medial posted heel, and with or without a metatarsal pad. Additional Reflex self-adhesive pads can be added to the orthotics to relieve pain from Morton's toe, sesamoiditis, and leg-length discrepancy. These orthotics are an alternative to custom-made orthotics. For more information

contact Apex Foot Health Industries, Inc. 170 Wesley Street, So. Hackensack, NJ 07606; (800) 526-2739; www.apexfoot.com.

- **Spenco Orthotic Arch Support** Spenco makes an Orthotic Arch Support that is heated in hot water and then shaped to your foot. They are available in either 3/4- or full-length. For more information contact Spenco Medical Corporation, PO Box 2501, Waco, TX 76702-2501; (800) 877-3626; www.spenco.com.

TacTape This unique tape comes on a roll that is 10 yards long by 1 3/4 inches wide. TacTape stretches in its width, but not in its length, helping to maintain the foots position in the shoe. The tape can be applied to any insole, orthotic, or the inside bottom of your shoe, boot, or sandal. It can also be used on the shoe's tongue or as a foot wrap directly on the skin or over the sock. Unaffected by water, the tape will hold its slip resistant features under any weather conditions. For more information contact TacLiner Footwear & Athletic Products, 14460 Cadillac Drive, San Antonio, TX 78248; (210) 479-5588; www.tacliner.com.

16

Nutrition for the Feet

In order to keep our feet healthy it is necessary to take care of them and to give them the nutrition they need. But then how many of us know what our feet really need?

Jillian Standish, a certified massage therapist, feels many runners simply don't think about using lotions or creams on their feet. Most of her clients are average runners who need the benefits of massage to enhance their running. Jillian focuses part of her massages on the feet since the lower leg muscles attach into the feet. As a pre-race conditioner, the massage helps loosen the muscles, often lengthening the runner's stride. As a post-race conditioner, she massages knots out of tired and stressed muscles.

In the summer when we are most active, our feet are often abused. Our feet become hard and callused or blistered by our multi-day hikes, long training runs on back-to-back days, cross-sport training, going barefoot, or wearing sandals without socks. We repeatedly stress our feet without giving them time to recover and to heal. In dry and cold weather our skin easily becomes too dry, resulting in cracks in the skin. When these cracks are deep they are called fissures and are often accompanied by calluses.

Use creams or lotions that help improve the skin's texture and tone by exfoliating dry and dead skin and allow newly rejuvenated skin to emerge. Some creams contain Alpha Hydroxy Acids which are all-natural substances found in fruits and sugar cane which generally speed up the exfoliation process. Ultrarunner Roy Pirrung uses flax oil products to keep his skin well conditioned.

A good testimonial for soft feet comes from race walker Dave Littlehales. He reports, "I used to think that tough, callused feet were the way to go. But after the '97 Vermont 100 where I developed huge full bottom of the feet blisters bilaterally, my podiatrist convinced me to go 100% in the other direction—soft and supple. Now I get a pedicure at least once a month smoothing out all calluses and rough spots. I also put creams on my feet on a daily basis. When I hit the trails or roads, I use foot powder. Things have improved greatly."

Massage is great for the feet. It helps increase circulation to injured areas and the increased blood supply helps speed recovery while reducing swelling. Sports massage focuses on releasing tight, contracted, overworked muscles used in your sport or activity and restoring them to their optimum condition. To do a self-massage of your feet, start by warming your feet in a bath or with warm, moist towels. Cross one leg over the other with the sole facing you. Use both thumbs to massage your feet in a deep, circular motion, working small areas at a time. Work from your toes toward your heel, and then to your ankle. Use various movements and pressure to find what feels best. All movement, and pressure, should be toward the heart—moving the old "stagnated" blood back to your heart. The use of massage oil or creams can help with the kneading of the skin and soften dry heels and calluses.

Long distance hiker Brick Robbins finds that after several months on the trail he has a hard time with "stuff" growing on his feet. He has solved this common problem by soaking his feet for 20 minutes in a solution of about a gallon of water and two to four ounces of providone-iodine every week or so. It keeps his "... feet from smelling too bad and seemed to kill the stuff that had started to grow under one of my big toes." Betadine will also work as an alternative to providone-iodine.

Products

FootSmart FootSmart carries a complete line of skin care products made for the feet. These products will help your feet feel softer and smoother. For information contact FootSmart Products, PO Box 922908, Norcross, GA 30010; (800) 870-7149; www.footsmart.com.

- Total Foot Recovery a cream/lotion with Alpha Hydroxy Acid and deep-penetrating Urethin to soften dry and callused feet.
- Callus Treatment Cream with Urethin to break down painful, hardened skin.
- Dr. D's Foot and Heel Cream with Tea Tree Oil, 10% Aloe Vera, and Vitamin E.
- Peppermint Pedicure Cream with a blend of Jojoba, Aloe Vera gel, and pure botanical extracts.
- Heel Treatment Cream with Urethin and Aloe Vera.
- Lansinoh Cream with 100% lanolin for superior moisturizing properties.
- Soothing Foot Balm with Witch hazel, Peppermint Oil, and Lavender Oil.
- A Callus File to reduce thick calluses.

A wide assortment of products is readily available at your local health food store or drug store. Below is a sampling of some products. Check your health food store or drug store for additional skin care products.

- Bioforce of America makes A. Vogel's Homeopathic 7 Herb Cream, a combination of herbs and oils in a natural base formulated to soften and smooth rough, dry, or cracked skin.
- Dr. Scholl's Rough Skin Removing Foot Cream.
- Flaxseed oil products containing sources of essential fatty acids for proper skin conditioning.
- FootTherapy Natural Mineral Foot Bath can be used to soak and soften corns and calluses.
- Neutrogena Foot Cream is a Norwegian formula that moisturizes and softens dry skin.

17

Hydration, Dehydration, & Sodium

A subject often overlooked is the effect to the skin of dehydration and the loss of important electrolytes. Long periods of physical exercise cause stress to the extremities as fluid accumulates in the hands and feet. Fingers and toes often swell as they retain fluid because of low blood sodium (hyponatremia). This causes foot problems as the soft, waterlogged tissues become vulnerable to the rubbing and pounding as we continue to run and hike.

Karl King, developer of the SUCCEED! Buffer/Electrolyte Caps points out that the maintenance of proper electrolyte levels will reduce swelling of hands and feet after many hours of exercise, and that will reduce "hot spots" and blisters on the feet. Make sure that you replace electrolytes, especially on long events. Drinking water or even sports drinks may not provide the proper replacement of sodium and other important electrolytes. The popular energy bars and gels may also be low in the electrolytes needed by the body.

It is important to understand, as ultrarunner Jay Hodde notes, "... 'proper hydration' and 'well hydrated' should not be used interchangeably. Being well hydrated with fluids says nothing about the sodium content of the fluid; both are important." As extra fluid accumulates in the tissues of the feet, from being well hydrated yet having low sodium, the likelihood of blister formation increases. When you become fluid-deficient, the skin loses its normal levels of water in the skin and loses its turgor. Then it easily rubs or folds over on itself that leads to blisters. The use of a sodium replacement product in prolonged physical activity can help in the prevention of blisters. Many athletes have found out the hard way, that simply drinking a fluid replacement drink often will not provide the necessary electrolytes in the proper concentrations that the body needs. SUCCEED! Electrolyte Caps, E-CAPS Endurolytes, and Thermotabs are products helpful in maintaining hydration and proper sodium levels.

Products

E-CAPS Endurolytes   E-CAPS makes Endurolytes as a Heat Stress Formula to counteract the effects of electrolyte depletion and imbalances of hot weather. The caps can be taken as a supplement or mixed in any fluid replacement drink. The Endurolyte caps contain calcium, magnesium, potassium, sodium chloride, L-Tyrosine, Vitamin B-6, and Manganese. For more information contact E-CAPS/Hammer Nutrition Ltd., PO Box 4010, Whitefish, MT 59937; (800) 336-1977; www.e-caps.com.

SUCCEED! Buffer/Electrolyte Caps
Ultrarunner and race director Karl King developed the SUCCEED! Buffer/Electrolyte Caps to provide electrolytes that are commonly found in blood plasma, in the proper proportions for hours of exercise. They are designed for individuals engaging in physical activities where they sweat heavily. The caps contain a chemical buffering system of sodium chloride, sodium bicarbonate, sodium citrate, sodium phosphate, and potassium chloride, that neutralizes the acids formed during heavy exercise. This both reduces nausea associated with exercise, particularly in the heat, and reduces swelling of hands and feet typically common after many hours of exercise. Karl reports positive results with the caps—a reduction in hot spots and blisters and reduced swelling in the hands and feet. They should not be used when water is in short supply. For more information contact UltraFit, W5297 Young Road, Eagle, WI 53119; (414) 495-3474; www.ultrafit-endurance.com.

Thermotabs   Thermotabs are buffered salt tablets that can be taken to prevent muscle cramps or heat prostration due excessive perspiration. Its active ingredients are sodium chloride and potassium chloride. Look for Thermotabs at your local drug store or pharmacy. Menley & James Laboratories, Inc. makes Thermotabs.

18

Anti-Perspirants for the Feet

The sweat glands on the soles of your feet normally produce small amounts of perspiration. According to the American Podiatric Medical Association the feet have approximately 250,000 sweat glands and produce as much as a pint of moisture each day. An increase in body temperature will increase the perspiration level. Some individuals have problems with excessive perspiration on their feet. The medical term "hyperhidrosis" refers to excessive moisture. This moisture often increases the chance of blisters. In these individuals, the use of an anti-perspirant on the feet may reduce the amount of perspiration. Reducing perspiration will help prevent the formation of blisters. David Zuniga is one runner who has found that the use of an anti-perspirant has helped his feet. He started using an anti-perspirant on the recommendation of his podiatrist and finds his feet stay "... dry as a bone."

Mike Palmer has worked at resolving blister problems related to sweaty feet. He wears sandals as much as he can to keep his feet dry during the day. A couple of weeks before a 100 miler, or an ultra of 50 miles or more, he uses alcohol at night to dry his feet. He finds coating his feet with Tincture of benzoin dries the skin as well as providing a protective coating. This has worked well for him. Before a 100-mile run, if the weather allows, he tries to walk about a mile barefoot about a month or so before the race in an attempt to further toughen the skin. Then before the run he uses an absorbent foot powder and puts dispensers of this powder in his drop bags at every point where he will make a sock change.

Mike also recommends frequent sock changes during long races—this is time consuming but it's better than trying to run on hot spots and blistered feet. For Mike, the moisture promotes blistering. Since using benzoin, the maceration (the whitish, flaky, condition of moist skin) has been eliminated and blistering is not so frequent or extensive.

In an interesting study, cadets attending the U.S. Military Academy were separated into two groups that used either an antiperspirant or placebo preparation. Each group was asked to apply their preparation for five consecutive nights before completing a 21-km hike. After the hike, only 21% of the cadets who reported using the antiperspirant preparation for at least three nights before the hike were diagnosed with foot blisters. The placebo group reported a 48% incidence of foot blisters. Joseph Knapik, ScD, the lead author of the study that appeared in the August 1998 issue of the *Journal of the American Academy of Dermatology* reported, "Blisters are usually minor problems, but they can cause great discomfort for the patient. Typically they only require simple first aid and a short period of limited activity. It is possible, however, for them to lead to more serious problems such as local or systemic infections." Researchers theorized that reducing sweating might reduce friction and consequently reduce blisters. The cadets applied the preparation to completely dry feet, up the ankle to the top of the boot line. Before the hike, each cadet was examined for existing foot conditions. Immediately after the hike, the feet of each cadet were inspected for blisters using the same criteria as the pre-hike examination. Researchers found that sweat reduction was a key mechanism for the reduction of blisters. While the antiperspirant was found to be very effective in reducing blisters, some side effects did occur. "Itching and rashes occurred in 57% of the antiperspirant group, but only 6% of the placebo group," Dr. Knapik stated. "This suggests that a large portion of the population may have problems with the antiperspirant used in the study. However, reducing the amount of the active compound or applying the antiperspirant every other night, rather than every night as the cadets did, may reduce the irritation."

The wearing of moisture wicking socks, frequent sock changes, and even shoe changes if the moisture is excessive, can help prevent problems. Several products offer a solution to this problem.

Products

Anti-Perspirants There are many anti-perspirants available in drug stores that can work on your feet. Check out the shelves at your local store and try one or two. Rich Schick recommends using Drysol, a prescription strength antiperspirant that is applied daily and after a couple days virtually eliminates all perspiration. Other have had success with Ban Roll-on.

DRYZ Insoles These insoles help the feet stay dryer and cooler while eliminating odor. The wicking sock liner transports the foot's perspiration and moisture into an inner layer of copolymer foam that absorbs and stores the moisture in a gel-like substance. The gelled moisture dissipates continuously throughout the day and completely when your shoes are removed. The odor killing agent ReSent and additional ingredients fight the growth of fungi and bacteria. Their sport insoles are engineered for enhanced comfort, cushion, and performance. For more information contact Dicon Technologies, 3-00 Banta Place, Fairlawn, NJ 07410; (877) 342-6685; www.dryz.com.

Foot Solution Foot Solution, by Onox, is a spray solution made to control excessive moisture and foot odor. A combination of mineral salts decreases excessive sweat and foot odor symptoms. The spray also helps reduce blistering and itching while repelling athlete's foot fungus. Ingredients include zinc chloride, deionized water, sodium chloride, sodium nitrate, boric acid, and sodium silco-fluoride. Be aware that the salt solution will sting if you have cuts or breaks in your skin. Foot Solution is available in a four-ounce spray pump. Foot Solution can be ordered through Healthy Legs & Feet Too, 6333 SW Macadam Ave., Suite 102, Portland, OR 97201; (888) 495-0105; www.healthy-legs.com.

Gold Bond Gold Bond is a medicated body powder that contains active ingredient zinc oxide as a skin protector and menthol to cool and relieve itching. Use the extra-strength powder for maximum benefits in absorbing excessive moisture. Gold Bond is made by Chattem, Inc. and is available through your local drug store and pharmacy.

Gordon's #5   Gordon Laboratories makes Gordon's #5, an aerosol foot powder which is helpful in reducing foot perspiration and foot odor. Gordon's #5 is available in a four-ounce size. Available only by special order through your local drug store, pharmacy, or podiatrist from Gordon Laboratories, 6801 Ludlow Street, Upper Darby, PA 19082; (800) 356-7870.

Zeasorb   The success of Zeasorb is in its super absorbent powder, which absorbs almost four times more moisture than plain talcum powder. Zeasorb contains talc, a highly absorbent polymer-carbohydrate acrylic copolymer, and microporous cellulose for super absorbency. This powder is very efficient and works without caking. The talc provides softness and lubrication to reduce friction and heat buildup. Their second powder, ZeasorbAF, with miconazole nitrate 2%, provides broad antifungal therapy and moisture control. Look for it at drug stores or order it through your local pharmacy. For more information contact Stiefel Laboratories, Inc., 255 Alhambra Circle, Coral Gables, FL 33134-7412; (305) 443-3800.

19

Gaiters

In 1989, before my third Western States 100-Mile Endurance Run, I knew I had to do something extra to help my feet. Since I was prone to blisters and the trail was known for its dust and rocks, I decided to make a pair of gaiters. My homemade gaiters are described below. While I realize the gaiters alone did not make the whole difference, I did lower my personal best time by 1 1/2 hours. The bottom line was that my feet were protected from the dust, grit, and rocks of the trail, and I had minimal problems.

Gaiters have proven themselves as functional trail running gear that all dedicated trail runners should have in their equipment bag. Hikers wearing low-top boots should consider the benefits of gaiters. Forming a barrier around the leg and the top of the shoe, gaiters keep rocks, dust, and water-borne grit from getting into socks or between the socks and shoe. Gaiters can mean the difference between finishing a trail run or long hike with feet in good shape or feet plagued with hot spots and blisters. Most gaiters close on the side or in the front with Velcro.

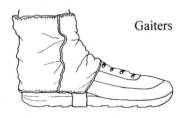

Gaiters

Raymond Zirblis wore women's knee highs over his shoes during the Marathon des Sables. The nylons stretched well, covered the whole shoe and up the leg, keeping sand and pebbles out, but the mesh was too open to keep dust out. While they tore and wore away, they stayed on through each day. Ray used a fresh pair each day, reporting that while not perfect, they worked better than most of the gaiter set-ups he saw there during the six days of the desert run.

Kent Holder tells of using the arms off an old nylon jacket with elastic sleeves. Cut the sleeves off about 6″ up the sleeve from the cuff. Simply pull the arms, elastic end first, onto your legs over your socks. The loose nylon covers the top of the shoes and Kent reports it keeps 100% of the usual trail debris from entering the shoe. With this type of gaiter, there are no straps, so changing your shoes and socks is a breeze. He suggests looking for old nylon jackets at your local thrift store. Rodney Hammons has found another way to get a gaiter effect. He wears a pair on knee-high type nylons under his Ultimax socks and then pulls the nylons down over the socks and tops of his shoes. Improvising can work wonders.

Repairing Gaiter Straps

The nylon straps or cords that come with most gaiters and goes under the shoes and boots will wear out over time as the trails and rocks take their toll. Wrapping the straps with duct tape can help extend their life span, then replace the tape when it wears through. There are several methods to replace the worn out straps.

The first method simply uses 1/4″ nylon cord. Cut the old strap 3/4″ from its attachments to the gaiter. Use a lighted match to slightly melt the ends of the straps to prevent fraying. Be careful to not touch the melted nylon until it cools. Punch a small hole in the middle of the 3/4″ section and use another lighted match to slightly melt the edges of the hole. Thread the nylon cord through the holes and knot securely so the length is the same as the old strap. Slightly melt the ends of the cord to avoid fraying.

Another method recommended by Mike Erickson uses swagged (pressed around the edges of the cable) 1/16″ stainless steel cable instead of the nylon cord—he reports these have held up for over five years. Put a piece of duct tape over the swagged ends. Mike also reports using thin nylon cord doused with superglue and then wrapped in a couple layers of duct tape. Others use tough shoe laces. Improvise to find other creative methods.

To replace the nylon strap itself, use the method recommended by ultrarunner Kirk Boisseree, using the following materials which are usually found in fabric stores: 1″ wide nylon webbing, size 24 (5/8″) large snaps (four sets of male and female pieces), and a snap installation tool. The snap tool can usually be found in craft or sewing stores. Make the new straps as follows.

- Using the old strap as a guide, cut two pieces of webbing the length of the old strap.
- At each end of the replacement straps, install a female snap. Use a center punch or a nail to make a hole in the center of the strap 3/4″ from each end. Push the snap through the hole and set the snap using the tool and following the instructions on the package. Repeat for all four snaps, making sure the snaps face the same way on each strap end.
- Install the male snaps on the old straps about 1/2″ to 3/4″ from the gaiter. Using the center punch and installation tool, center the male snap in the hole, facing the outside of the shoe and set the snap.
- Cut the center out of the worn strap by cutting about 1/2″ from the new snaps.
- Use a lighted match to slightly melt the ends of the straps to prevent fraying. Be careful to not touch the melted nylon until it cools.
- Snap on the new straps and check for a proper fit.

Products

Homemade Gaiters   Homemade gaiters for running shoes or boots can be made out of a pair of regular white crew socks. Pull the socks on your feet and with a scissors, cut the socks around the foot at the top of the shoe line. Toss out the foot portions. Fold the top of the sock down on itself so the folded down top covers the top of the shoe. Make a small hole in this folded down top at the back of the shoe and just to the rear of each upper shoe lace eyelet. Make similar holes in the shoe. Through the shoe hole place a plastic twist tie from a loaf of bread or similar package. By twisting the ties through these matching holes you have effectively covered the top of the shoes. Undo the twist ties to change shoes or socks while leaving the sock gaiter on your leg.

MiniGators   MiniGators are designed to be "just-big-enough" to fit over the top of boots and shoes. Made from a stretchy, flexible Spandura material, this one-piece design is pulled onto the foot over the sock with the gaiter bottom stretching over the top of the shoe and attaching to the shoe lace with a hook. A flat lace runs under the shoe's instep and ties on both sides of the shoe. There are four models: the Trail Racer, designed for trail running and adventure racing; the Arizona, for hiking and backpacking in hot, dry climates; the Original Hiker, for a variety of environments including wet climates; and the Rainier, for mountaineering and winter sports. The first two are lightweight and breathable, the latter two are waterproof but breathable. For more information contact MiniGators, 4730 21st Avenue NE, Suite 109, Seattle, WA 98105; (888) 539-3923; www.minigators.com.

Outdoor Research   Outdoor Research makes three gaiter styles appropriate for running and hiking. The Flex-Tex Low Gaiter is a one-size-fits-all, made from stretchy Spandura fabric, is suited for hiking boots or running shoes. The Rocky Mountain Low Gaiters are made from vapor permeable uncoated packcloth in one-size-fits-all. The Rocky Mountain High Gaiters are available in either Gore-Tex fabric or packcloth in small, medium, large, and extra-large. All gaiters open in the front with Velcro, have an eyelet on either side for a lace that goes under the shoe's arch, and a metal hook that fastens to a shoelace. For more information contact Outdoor Research, 2203 1st Avenue South, Seattle, WA 98134-1424; (888) 4OR-GEAR; www.orgear.com. Sells through distributors only, no online sales.

RaceReady Trail Gaitors   The folks from RaceReady, who make the pocketed running shorts, also make good Trail Gaitors for running shoes and low-top hiking boots. Made in a combination of colors from quick drying and breathable Supplex nylon, these gaiters have a "space-age tough" cord that goes under the shoe's arch. The cord allows for a custom fit for your type and size of shoe. These fasten with the usual Velcro closure on the outside of the shoe. Sizes are small, medium, large, and extra-large. These could be used on other hiking boots by lengthening the strap. For more information contact RaceReady, PO Box 251065, Glendale, CA 91225-1065; (800) 537-6868; www.raceready.com.

Western States 100 Trail Gaiters The Western States 100-Mile Endurance Run offers running shoe trail gaiters. These gaiters are made of nylon Condura fabric with a light urethane coating. A snap on each side of the gaiter attaches to the nylon strap that goes under the shoe and is also held in place with a Velcro strip. An extra pair of straps is included with each pair of gaiters. These gaiters are available in medium, large, and extra-large sizes and can also be worn with many of the low-top hiking boots either as is or by lengthening the strap. For more information contact the Western States 100-Mile Endurance Run, 242 Hartnell Place, Sacramento, CA 95825; Greg Soderlund, gsoderlund@juno.com; www.ws100.com.

20

Lacing Options

Some runners have problems with laces causing friction and pressure. After a long run or hike, some runners and hikers experience bruising over the instep where the laces tie. Laces can be adjusted to fine-tune the fit of the shoe or boot and to relieve pressure over the instep. The lacing variations described below can make a shoe fit better and allow for needed spacing in the tongue area or provide for better heel control. The conventional method of lacing, criss-cross to the top of the shoe, works best for the majority of people. In the illustrations, dotted lines show where laces are hidden from view.

Flat feet, high arches or not enough support in the arches, narrow or wide feet, and heel control problems can be helped, to varying degrees, by lacing techniques. Several of the lacing techniques described below work best with shoes having alternating eyelets spaced apart, not up and down in a straight line.

For narrow feet, use the eyelets farthest from the tongue of the shoe. This will bring up the sides of the shoe for a tighter fit across the top of the foot. This method works on shoes with variable width eyelets.

For wide feet, use the eyelets closest to the tongue of the shoe. This gives the foot more space by giving more width across the lace area. This method works

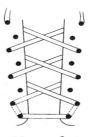

Narrow feet

best on shoes with variable width eyelets. An alternative method is to pass back under the parallel segment of lace between the first and second eyelet to create a half hitch knot, this prevent the lace across the first eyelets from getting tighter as you run.

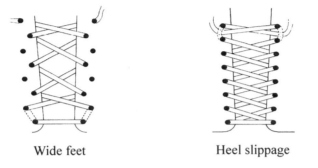

Wide feet   Heel slippage

For heel slippage or problems, use every eyelet, making sure that the area closest to the heel is tied tightly while less tension is used near the toes. When you have reached the next to the last eyelet on each side, thread the lace through the top eyelet of the same side, making a small loop. Then thread the opposite lace through each opposite loop before tying the laces together at the top.

For high arches, lace the shoes so the laces go straight across. After lacing the bottom two eyelets on the outer side to the inner two eyelets, lace up two eyelets on the same inner side and cross over to the outer side. Lace through these two eyelets and move up two eyelets on the same outer side. Continue this alternating method until one set of eyelets is left. Now lace up to the top eyelets on each side.

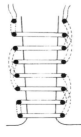 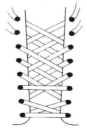

High arches   High arch alternative

An alternative method for high arches is to lace one lace through the first two bottom eyelets and then every other eyelet to the top. A second lace is threaded through the remaining eyelets. This allows tighter lacing at the ball of the foot and the ankle while the mid-foot is laced looser. With this method, quick adjustments are easily made for uphills and downhills.

For a narrow heel and wide forefoot use one pair of laces per shoe. Lace one through the bottom half of the eyelets tied loosely. Lace the other through the top half of the eyelets tied more tightly than the bottom lace. Another option is to lace the first few loops loosely, tie a knot, and then lace the rest of the way up the shoe.

For foot pain, lace as normal for your foot type and skip the eyelets over the pain area.

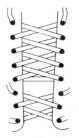

Narrow heel and
wide forefoot

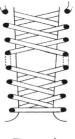

Foot pain

For toenail problems or corns, lace down from the top eyelet opposite the problem toe to the bottom eyelet on the side of the problem toe, leaving enough end to tie the laces together. Then from the bottom up, side-to-side until the top eyelet is reached. This method creates an upward tension on the bottom eyelet over the problem toe, relieving pressure.

To maintain a consistent lace pressure at the toes, lace the bottom eyelets as usual. Then lock the lace in place by looping the lace around and back through the same eyelet. Continue lacing as normal. Locking the lace at the second or third eyelet can modify this technique. This allows you to tie the laces as tight as you want above the lock while keeping the laces as loose as desired below the lock.

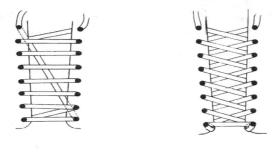

Toenail problems or corns   Constant toe pressure

In all cases rather than double knotting gather the loops and lace ends and tuck them through one or two of the cross strands towards the toe of the shoe. This prevents laces from coming untied as effectively as double knotting and is much easier to untie. Also when running through brush it keeps the laces from getting snagged or picking up debris.

Several lacing products work well for running shoes some boots, actually any type of shoe. Easy-Laces have been around for over 20 years and are a favorite with many athletes. Air-Laces are a newer lacing concept that also works well. These products replace the normal shoelaces and end the problem of laces coming untied or broken. Experiment with stretch laces to find the most comfortable degree of lace tightness that does not cause undo pressure on the instep and yet controls the heel. A product that can help with instep irritations is a tongue cushion.

Products

Air-Lace Shoelaces   Air-Lace Shoelaces are made for all types of footwear. The laces are made of a thin, stretchable latex based tube. The laces are fed through the shoe eyelets from the top to the bottom and joined at the bottom with a connector. This allows you to slide on your shoes or mid- and low-top boots. There are no knots or bows. These laces eliminate the problem of pressure on the foot where the shoelace knots. Air-Laces are available in a variety of colors. They may not work for high-top shoes or boots. To order these laces contact Netstuff.com at (800) 472-0757; www.netstuff.com/airlace/index.htm.

Easy Laces   Easy Laces Lockable Shoelaces are a great alternative to shoelaces for running shoes and most hiking boots. The lace is a stretchy elastic cord with an interlocking lock where the usual bow is tied. The foot is slipped into the shoe or boot without releasing the lock, or the lock can be released to open the shoe further. The laces are available in a myriad of colors. For those not wanting the lock at the instep, cross the right lace over and under the shoe and the through the lock. This moves the lock to the side of the shoe. The Stretch-Lace Company makes Easy Laces. For more information contact Stretch-Lace Co, PO Box 902, Norwood, MA 02062; (800) 572-3247; www.easy-laces.com.

Hapad Tongue Cushion   Hapad makes a Tongue Cushion that prevents rubbing and comforts shoe irritations at the instep. If you have narrow heels, it also holds the foot back into the heel of the shoe for a better fit. The coiled, spring-like wool fibers provide firm and resilient support. The pad attaches to the underside of the tongue of the shoe. For more information contact Hapad Inc., PO Box 6, 5301 Enterprise Blvd., Bethel Park, PA 15102; (800) 544-2723; www.hapad.com.

21

Changing Your Shoes and Socks

On long runs, determine how often you will change your shoes and socks. Ultrarunner Dave Scott changes his shoes four to five times in a 100-mile trail race. At each change he reapplies more Vaseline to his toes. Aid stations that are accessible to crew support or aid stations that have your drop bags are the best choices. On a 24-hour run consider having additional half and full size larger shoes available may save your feet.

When possible, change your socks and/or shoes before problems develop. Dry skin is more resistant to blister formation than skin that has been softened by moisture. Trail running and hiking often makes for wet shoes and boots which become dirt-caked. Shoes and socks should be changed as soon as possible after getting wet. Depending on the event, you may choose to change at pre-determined points or pre-determined times. This may be as many as four to five times in a long 100-mile run. At these times, the feet should be inspected for problems and treatments made. Power and/or lubricants should be reapplied when changing socks.

While shoes and socks do dry out after a stream crossing or in rain, continuing to run or hike may cause the skin on your feet to become overly soft and tender and more prone to blisters. Softening of the skin, called maceration, can cause skin over and around blisters to separate. Where the blister is already ruptured, the skin then opens up. When the skin has been wet for long periods of time, it is not uncommon, when removing socks, to find the skin as shriveled as a prune and the skin separating. The use of high technology oversocks to keep the feet dry can help reduce maceration and blisters. Refer to the *High-Technology Oversocks* section on page 72 for information on these socks.

As difficult as it becomes, you must take the time to properly manage your feet, or your feet will manage you as problems develop and you are reduced to a slow, limping walk. When you are close to an age-group win, a personal best, simply finishing within the time limit, or reaching a specific trail destination, the three to ten minutes necessary for foot care may seem like a lifetime. Only you can make the decision on taking the time to care for your feet. I have seen many runners take off their shoes and socks to reveal skin which fall off the bottom of their feet. Not small pieces but enough to cover half their foot! It cannot be emphasized enough—take the time necessary to manage your feet or they will manage you.

Runners may choose to carry an extra pair of socks and a small foot care kit in a fanny pack, allowing for road or trailside foot care as necessary. Hikers need to carry a foot care kit as part of a first-aid kit. They should wash their dirty socks daily and dry them on the back of their packs. Some hikers will wisely choose to change socks every three hours. If possible, take a few minutes for a short five to ten minutes soak in a cold stream or lake to refresh your tired feet. Before putting stream washed socks back on your feet, turn them inside out and fluff up the fabric to restore some of their loft.

In extremely cold weather, it is important to keep the feet dry and warm. Socks and footwear that are too tight can cause constriction and impede circulation. Changing from wet into dry socks helps keep the feet warm. The use of moisture-wicking socks also is helpful. See the section *High-Technology Oversocks* on page 72 for information on these socks that can help ward off cold.

Frostbite can happen to toes, but is avoidable. Frostbite requires freezing temperature. Constriction can be caused by tight shoes, too many pairs of socks, and shoelaces toed to tight. Whether using running shoes or boots, one can easily get frostbite in a dry set of shoes or boots that are tied too tight and not allowing proper blood circulation. Good circulation will help keep your feet warm.

Dehydration makes athletes more susceptible to frostbite. The use of anti-perspirants to control moisture can help. Symptoms of frostbite include cold, pain, dulling of the pain (frostnip), numbness, a doughy or wooden look, and pain on rewarming. If you suspect frostbite, do not wash away the skin's natural oils. If your feet are frostbitten, do not rewarm them if you must walk to help, but wait until medical help is available.

22

Teamwork and Crew Support

There may be times when you are involved in a team sport or a sport that utilizes a crew. Adventure racing is typically done as a team. Backpacking and hiking, while not team sports, may be done as a group. Crew support is found in ultramarathon events, adventure racing, and team sports: football, soccer, etc. What needs to be thought out ahead of your race or activity is what kind of planning is necessary and what are the responsibilities of each team or crew member. First, a look at teamwork is helpful.

Teamwork

Anytime you are with a group, teamwork is vital. You are only as strong as your weakest member and as fast as your slowest member. If you have a crew supporting you and you need footcare, can any crew member manage your feet—or only one? Do team members know how to care for each others feet as well as their own?

For adventure racing this is of particular importance. As you train and race, your team will learn from each other's strengths and build on each other's weaknesses. It may sound easy, but this aspect is rated as one of the most complex and difficult of all adventure racing components. Each team member must have some degree of skill at all of the disciplines—including footcare. The same can be said for all members of a backpacking or hiking. A story of one team's experience during one adventure race will illustrate this point.

Patty Hintz, a member of Team R.E.A.R. participated in a two-day adventure race in the Shasta Trinity Alps. She recalls, "The mileage for the running section was about 35 miles and one of my teammates had a problem with blisters. Being an experienced ultrarunner I brought along extra Spenco 2nd Skin. When she said blisters, I had no idea we were talking both heels, both forefeet, and multiple toes on each foot! We had three different types of tape to put over the 2nd Skin. I first tried moleskin—but a few miles later it was off. Next was cloth tape, but it did not hold either. Finally, I remembered the duct tape in our team's mandatory gear. I don't know how she managed but she said her feet felt 100% better. She was able to continue the race and the duct tape never came off."

This story is important in that Patty had anticipated foot problems and was prepared. She knew the value of 2nd Skin and knew how to apply tape to the feet. She also knew how to improvise. If she had been on a team where no one how to properly drain blisters and tape over them, they may not have finished the two-day event.

Patty tells that, "Later we talked about what caused the blisters? She had great socks made for running to reduce friction. Her shoes had plenty of break in time and fit her feet properly. I personally think it was not enough experience with time on her feet. I honestly feel if your shoes fit you properly, you wear appropriate socks, you buy the right type of shoe for the way you run, and you spend time breaking a new pair of shoes in before you race in them; blisters are going to come until your feet have enough distance and time to toughen up. Until then I'm a firm believer in duct tape and 2nd Skin. As far as my teammate's feet, I'm happy to say they healed very quickly about a week."

Planning for Footcare

People participating in the same activity or teams would be wise to sit down before an event, particularly if it is your first or second event together, or your first multi-day event, and talk about footcare. Who has the most footcare experience? What is the best way to prepare your feet—pre-event taping, toughening your skin, better socks, and/or better fitting shoes? As Patty asks, "Does each member have enough time on their feet to toughen them for the distance?" What is the best method to use when fixing blisters? How about really big blisters? What is the minimum amount of footcare knowledge expected of each person? What footcare gear will you carry and how much of each item? Footcare kits are useless if only one person know how to use the materials in them. Who then will fix that person's feet if problems develop? And who will manage the team's feet if that person is injured or has to be pulled from the race?

Team Responsibilities

Whatever you carry in a footcare kit, know how to use each item. Each member of the team should know how to tape their feet to prevent and fix blisters. Each team member should work at finding what is best for their feet—lubricants or powders, two pairs of socks or one pair, double layer socks or single layer, how to lace their shoes for specific foot problems, and how to find the best fitting shoes for their feet. It is the responsibility of the whole team to be sure each member is adequately trained in proper footcare. It can mean the difference between a good race and in just finishing—or even not finishing.

Crew Support

If you will be participating in an event where you have crew support to help you at aid stations make sure to discuss foot care issues with them before the event. Let them know if there will be shoe or sock changes at particular aid stations, and if so, what specific shoes or socks you will want. Let them know all of the following.

- How to take your shoes and socks off to avoid making any foot problems worse.
- How to put new shoes and socks back on.
- What powders and/or lubricants you use and where on your feet you use them.
- How tight you like your shoes tied, and whether you use single or double knots.
- How you want to deal with hot spots, blisters, toenails, or other unique problems.

Practice this with your crew at home, well in advance of the run. By trial and error find what works and what doesn't work. It is important to know the amount of time these activities will take.

When arriving in the aid station, let them know what you need for your feet. Advise them of any hot spots or blisters. Never let them pull shoes off your feet without proper unlacing. This action, however unintentional, can rupture a blister or cause increased pain to already hurting feet. A shoehorn can be a lifesaver to easily slide the heel out of and into the back of the shoe without too much pressure on sore and tender heels.

23

Multi-Day Events

Multi-day races are a challenge to even the experienced athlete. There may be changing weather conditions, water from rain, wind and cold, or heat and humidity. No two multi-day events will be the same. You must be prepared whatever is thrown at you. Proper pre-event planning with your shoes, socks, and footcare kit, along with all your other gear, is crucial. Whether you are doing a 100-mile trail run that takes 40 hours, a six-day road race, or a three-day adventure race, you must take care of your feet from the start. Some suggestions are appropriate for road races but not for trail races or events that are a mix of road and trail. Modify the ideas to fit your event.

Dan Brannen, an experienced multi-day ultrarunner, has several ideas for the problem of swollen feet in multi-day races. He has learned, "In the latter stages of multi-days on tracks or road loops, my enlarging feet felt best with no socks and open-toe running shoes. The biggest cause of serious swelling during a multi-day is, ironically, being off your feet. The best way to avoid really troublesome foot swelling is to stay on the track as much as possible. Any rest breaks longer than a few hours are just going to make your feet bigger. Forget icing, elevation, and rest during the race. Their effect will be inconsequential. Dan also recommends, when traveling home after the event (especially when flying), wearing sandals over socks. Or, wear your shoes loose and untied—even when walking through the airport.

Peter Bakwin, a veteran multi-day trail runner, observed a multi-day race with the following comments, "I also noticed a lot of the multi-day runners had the toes cut out of their shoes. We camped next to one runner and she had several pair like that and her shoes were probably two sizes bigger than you would normally use. She also changed her shoes and socks frequently, rotating socks to get dry ones. I also noticed that a lot of the six-day guys were using very thin nylon stockings under their regular socks." Trauma shears make short work of cutting shoes and should be available at any race that has medical support. These shears are a good all-purpose tool for your multi-day foot repair kit.

Ray Zirblis writes from the experience of 24-hour and multi-day stage races. He knows first-hand that foot swelling can trouble racers. He shares, "After the Orlander Park 24-Hour, my feet are typically quite swollen for four or five days. Air and auto travel home is always excruciating. Once home, I keep a bucket of ice water by my bed and every couple of hours, when those 'dogs begin to bark,' I get up and soak them. During my first 100-milers, I had a house by a stream and would sleep out by the bank so I could roll over and dunk them periodically."

When I did a 72-hour road race, I learned that a quick 20-minute nap every six hours helped me stay sharp. From 12 hours on, I took these quick "cat naps" for the remaining 60 hours. During my naps, I slightly elevated my feet—with my shoes off.

Multi-day events are unique and will affect each athlete's feet differently. It is wise to know your options before the event. Some tips to consider for multi-day events include the following.

- Cut the toes out of your shoes (if the location and terrain allow)
- Frequent icing
- Elevate your feet when resting
- Immersing your feet in ice water during occasional break periods
- Have extra shoes a size or two larger than normal, with interchangeable insoles
- Rotate your socks to keep your feet as dry as possible

- Use different thicknesses of socks
- Use anti-inflammatory medications
- Change shoes and socks frequently
- Use very thin nylon stockings under regular socks

Going into a multi-day event without knowing the best way to care for your feet and how to fix blisters or a turned ankle can spell disaster. Practice before your event and as the preceding chapter suggests, if you have a team or crew, or are on a team or crew, learn everything you can about how to take care of and fix feet.

Part Three

Treatments

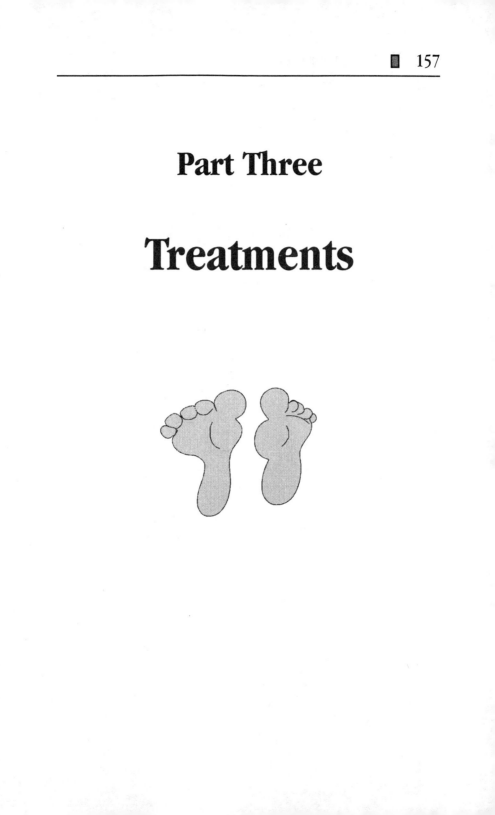

24

Treatments to Fix Your Feet

"The 4ᵗʰ Law of Running Injuries:
Virtually All Running Injuries Are Curable.
Only a minute fraction of true running injuries are not entirely
curable by quite simple techniques ..."
Tim Noakes, MD, *The Lore of Running.*[18]

No matter how hard we try to prevent problems with our feet, there may come a time when repair is needed. Then you have to become reactive. This section explains how to fix foot problems that typically develop. It is always best to know how to fix problems before they develop. Beginning a long trail run or a multi-day hike without preparing for the possibility of blisters, a sprained ankle, or other potential injury is foolhardy. One or two unexpected blisters at the wrong time can spell the end to a long anticipated event.

The Marathon des Sables is an extreme race, a six-day, self-supported race in the Moroccan desert that treats runners to 150-miles of sand, sand, and more sand, 200-foot sand dunes, rocky roads with small odd-shaped stones, heat that sucks the moisture out of your skin, and winds and sandstorms that torment every inch of your being. Robert Nagle, a highly experienced Eco-Challenge adventure racer, ran the race in 1997 and had only one blister. He commented that, "Many of the participants have neither the experience or knowledge of foot care for ultras—so they suffer mightily." The name of the game is to plan ahead to finish well and with healthy feet. If you don't, you are at a disadvantage right from the start.

Dave Covey, an experienced ultrarunner, in 1996 participated in a competitive and challenging 25-day 600 km wilderness trek across Western Australia which stressed his feet beyond his wildest imagination. While working in a walking and backpacking shoe store, he studied the different types of boots and selected a nylon and leather boot with a Gore-Tex fabric interior. The combination of high temperatures, long pants, and wearing heavy-duty nylon gaiters to protect his legs from the spiny vegetation made his legs sweat constantly. With his feet always wet, and the very uneven and rocky terrain, his feet were subject to extreme punishment. Changing into dry wicking style socks every two hours helped for the first two days. By the third day blisters had developed on the bottoms of his toes. Moleskin simply would not adhere to the wet skin. By the end of the eighth day he rested his feet for a few days to try to dry out the blisters. He then used Betadine and duct tape on the toes. By the eighteenth day, the skin finally began to callous over and during the last six days of the trek he did not have to use any tape. Dave gave his boots high marks for comfort, realizing the blisters were caused by other factors.

When your feet are tired, there are several ways for you to help them feel better. When changing socks, stopping for lunch, or whenever possible, take a few minutes and massage your feet and check for any hot spots. A short soak in an icy stream or in a bucket of cold water can revitalize tired feet. When you sit down to change socks or shoes after being on your feet for any great length of time, elevating your feet above the level of your heart will help reduce swelling of the feet. While hiking or on adventure races, try to wash your feet with soap and water at least once per day, preferably in the evening.

The chapters in this section provide information on dealing with foot problems common to runners, hikers, and adventure racers. Included are descriptions of the problem, ways to treat the problem, products that can help relieve or solve the problem, and, in some cases, exercises to strengthen the affected areas. Read the chapters that pertain to your injury history and try the treatments and products to find those that resolves your problems.

25

Hot Spots

Most runners experience hot spots in the areas where they are susceptible to blisters forming. The area will become sore and redness appears—thus the name "hot spot." There may also be a stinging or burning sensation. Around the reddened area will be a paler area that enlarges inward to where the skin is being rubbed.[19] The area becomes elevated as the surface skin is lifted as it fills with fluid. The hot spot has then become a blister.

Treatments

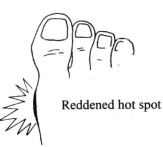

Reddened hot spot

We must deal with these hot spots before they become blisters. By the time the hot spot has developed enough to be felt, protection is necessary. Use your choice of one of the tapes or blister care products described in this book to protect the area. If you have used lubricants or powders on your feet, wipe the area with an alcohol wipe before applying tape, adhesive felt, or moleskin. Take the time to deal with hot spots as you feel them develop. Continuing to run or hike on them will only make them worse. They usually then turn into blisters which are harder to treat.

Examine your shoes or boots to determine whether you can modify them to remove the pressure point causing the problem.

You may have to make a slit or cut out a small section in the side or toe of the shoe. Start with a small cut or hole and enlarge it as necessary.

26

Blisters

Basically put, blisters are an injury. And as we all know, blisters can be painful. One blister, in a sensitive place on the foot, can easily ruin an otherwise good day. Blisters have often destroyed months of training and hundreds of dollars spent on a major event. Several blisters can drain your energy and reduce a runner to a walker or a hiker to a plodder, which in turn tends to create more blisters, which then slows forward motion even more. Too many athletes fail to educate themselves about blister prevention and how to do adequate blister care. Many runners and hikers think blisters are unavoidable and simply a part of the running or hiking process. Sometimes I think we should offer an award to those with the biggest blisters! Yet, somehow, when you remove a runner's shoe at the Highway 49 aid station at Western States and the skin falls off of half of each foot, you realize the runner should not get an award, but an education on good foot care.

Some athletes claim to have feet with skin as soft as a baby's bottom while others take pride in having thick calluses on the bottom of their feet. Both may claim to never blister and yet on another day, in a different race or activity with different conditions and variables, both may blister. Kevin

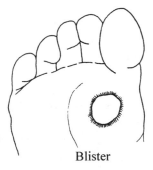

Blister

Setnes keeps telling us, "We are each an experiment of one." We need to remember that our feet change. Other blister-causing factors also change race to race—weather conditions, a lack of foot conditioning through training, the body's hydration level, the length of the race, running biomechanics as the runner reacts to a sore hamstring or tight quads, for example—all contribute to potential problems.

Blisters come in a variety of sizes. They start small, from a hot spot, and can continue to grow larger until they are treated. One blister may not seem like much, but suddenly you have two, and then, maybe three. Multiply the pain of one well-placed blister times three or four, like some people get, and you and imagine how severe a seemingly minor problem can become.

When he did the 1992 Trans-America, ultrarunner A.J. Howie described his blisters as "... pepperoni pizza blisters," large enough to make the Guinness Book of World Records. Blisters can also become major nightmares. John Supler, participating in the Marathon des Sables, a 155-mile six-day stage race across the Moroccan Sahara desert reported, "When I came in my feet were shredded like noodles. And when I woke up, my foot was stuck to my silk sheet, with a pool of yellow pus underneath it, leaking out."

The time and conditions required for blisters to develop will vary from individual to individual. Runners and hikers tend to get either "downhill" blisters on the toes and forefoot caused by friction while going downhill and "uphill" blisters on the heels and over the Achilles tendons caused by friction while going uphill. Blisters on the heel can also mean the heel cup is too wide. Blisters on the top or front of the toes or the outsides of the outer toes can indicate friction in the toe box.

Blisters 101

A basic understanding of how blisters are formed is necessary to successfully treat them. Remember the triangle mentioned earlier (p.55)? The factors of heat, friction, and moisture around the triangle contribute to the formation of blisters. Studies have shown that the foot inside the shoe or boot is exposed to friction at many sites as it experiences motion from side to side, front to back, and up and down. These friction sites also change during the activity as the exercise intensity, movement of the sock, and flexibility of the shoe or boot changes.[20]

The outer epidermis layer of skin receives friction that causes it to rub against the inner dermis layer of skin. This friction between the layers of skin causes a blister to develop. As the outer layer of the epidermis is loosened from the deeper layers, the sac in between becomes filled with lymph fluid. A blister has then developed. If the blister is deep or traumatically stressed by continued running or hiking, the lymph fluid may contain blood. When the lymph fluid lifts the outer layer of epidermis, oxygen and nutrition to this layer is cut off and it becomes dead skin. This outer layer is easily burst. The fluid then drains and the skin loses its natural protective barrier. The underlying skin is raw and sensitive. At this point the blister is most susceptible to infection.

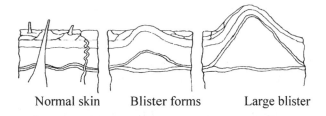

Normal skin   Blister forms   Large blister

The friction against whatever is touching the skin causes the friction between the layers of skin. As identified earlier, the majority of foot problems can be traced back to socks, powders, and lubricants—or the lack of them. In order to prevent blisters, friction must be reduced. Friction can be reduced in three main ways: 1) wearing double-layer socks or one inner and one outer sock, 2) keeping the feet dry by using powders, or 3) by using a lubricant to reduce chafing. It has been found that rubbing moist skin tends to produce higher friction than does rubbing skin that is either very dry or very wet.[21] Since the skin blisters more easily when soft and moist, it is important to understand the value of moisture-wicking socks coupled with knowing whether powders and/or lubricants are best for your feet and how to use them. Eliminating pressure points caused by poor-fitting insoles and/or ill-fitting shoes can also reduce friction. As stated earlier, examine your shoes or boots to try to eliminate the pressure point causing the blister. Cut slits or holes in the shoes as necessary.

Since your footwear causes blisters, the healing process truly begins when these are removed. If you have the option of a day's layover in camp without shoes and socks, this can speed the healing process and get you back on your feet faster and feeling better. Wearing sandals without socks exposes the blister to the air, which aids in healing.

Try to avoid getting blisters on top of existing blisters. When your skin is healing, protect or cushion the tender area.

Blisters Yesterday, Today, and Tomorrow

The problem, which most of us face at one time or another is that what has worked for us in the past, is no longer working. Ultrarunner Marv Skagerberg candidly warns "Caveat pedis, or let the toes beware. I have completely solved the blister problem 12 times by perfecting various methods that allow me to run for 24 hours and up, blister free. However the next time out with the exact same method, I have plenty of blisters." He has found that a combination of tincture of benzoin and silicone cream is by far the best for his feet. (See the section *Extreme Blister Prevention and Care* on page 177 for his method). Yesterday's method may have worked for years. Today's method may work for years. But then again, as Marv warns, it may not.

Tony Burke recalls the way he approached his 1996 backpack of the 211-mile John Muir Trail in California's Sierra Nevada.

> I had hoped that 15 years as a long distance runner and backpacker had eliminated the element of surprise in regards to foot problems and their treatment. I was wrong.
> The first day of my 17-day hike required an additional 11-mile

climb to the trailhead atop Mt. Whitney's 14,500-foot summit. On the way up, both heels started to blister. A little early in the trip I thought, but not unexpected. I immediately applied my favorite remedy, "2nd Skin." This was to become a daily ritual. The 2nd Skin would ease the soreness and keep the wounds reasonably clean but the Adhesive Knit that held it in place could not withstand the rigors of such a brutal, rocky trail and the blisters worsened to over an inch in diameter. Every step was painful, distracting me from the trail's beautiful surroundings. Soon, I ran out of Adhesive Knit, and resorted to that trusty standby, "duct tape." This kept the dressings in place longer, but, after clambering up and over yet another 12,000-foot pass, it too would slip. Then I got a rash from the tape's adhesive and smaller blisters from the tape's edges.

At my resupply point, nine days into the trip, I stocked up on 2nd Skin and duct tape, and padded the heel cups of my two-year old "broken-in" boots with moleskin and more duct tape. This stopped any future heel blistering but pushed my toes forward in the boots just enough to cause a whole new set of foot problems for the final leg of my trip. Some days it just isn't worth getting out of bed!

Tony's years of running and backpacking gave him a good base of experience—but he was venturing into new territory. The length of the trip, the rugged terrain, and the heavier backpack put added stresses on his feet.

The late ultrarunner Dick Collins used to have problems with blisters. After trying recommendations from others, including tape, he formed his own conclusion. Dick learned that "... anything other than socks on my feet will over time become an irritant." He used only Vaseline on his feet and wore synthetic socks. Having completed 1037 races, including 238 ultras, he found what worked for him and stuck to it. Like Dick, we each need to learn what works for us and be open to trying new ideas and products that could help keep our feet healthy.

We have no guarantee that what works one-day will work another day. Damon Lease experienced the frustration many athletes face when they do everything the same as they have done before and still blister. By mile 20 of a 50-mile race he was feeling hot spots on his toes. By mile 38 he was reduced to a painful walking state. At the 42.2-mile aid station he made the difficult decision to stop. Damon said, "I did nothing different in this race than any other ultra." He had used the same shoe and sock combination in other ultras but this course was steeper with "... more loose rocks and rough footing than the others." It happens. The trick is to play with all the variables in training to find what works best for your feet. Then be prepared with additional options in your gear bag.

General Blister Care

From the perspective of runners and hikers, the goal of blister treatments is to make the foot comfortable since often running or hiking must continue. Bryan P. Bergeron, MD, in an article "A Guide to Blister Management,"[22] identifies four therapeutic goals of blister management as: avoiding infection, minimizing pain and discomfort, stopping further blister enlargement, and maximizing recovery. He recommends all blister treatments be considered with these four goals in mind.

Avoiding infection

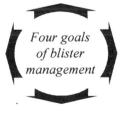

Stopping further blister enlargement

Four goals of blister management

Minimizing pain and discomfort

Maximizing recovery

For years, normal blister care has been gauze, moleskin, and Vaseline. Anyone can slap on a piece of moleskin and slather on some Vaseline and hope for the best. But to really fix a blister so you can continue running or hiking is an art. Walking among the podiatrists at the finish line of a marathon or ultra, one finds most blister care practices incorporate these three materials.

The time-honored method of blister care uses moleskin to protect the blister. If the blister is intact, cut a piece of moleskin about 1/2″ to 3/4″ larger around than the blister, with a hole slightly larger than the blister in the center. Press it on the skin around the blister and put an antibiotic ointment, Bag Balm, or medicated Vaseline in the hole over the blister. The final step is to tape a piece of gauze over the moleskin. Adding a piece of adhesive knit or tape over the gauze will help hold it in place.

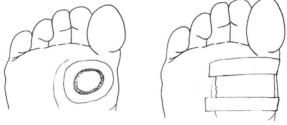

Moleskin with hole cut out for blister

Gauze over moleskin

Alternatives to moleskin are adhesive felt, one of the tapes identified earlier, or Spenco Pressure Pads. You can also use one of the tapes or Spenco Skin Knit in place of the gauze.

Basic Blister Repair

If the above treatment does not help or if you must continue running or hiking, time should be taken to repair a blister before it enlarges and ruptures. Dr. Bergeron recommends draining the blister prior to applying a dressing when it is in a weight-bearing area and larger than 0.8″ in diameter.[23] Use an alcohol wipe or hydrogen peroxide to clean the skin around the blister. Then use a pin or needle, flame-sterilized by heating with a match (avoid soot on the tip), to lance two to four puncture holes in a row in the blister. Making a single large hole increases the possibility of the blister roof shearing off when running or hiking must continue. Make the puncture holes on the side of the blister where ongoing foot pressure will push out additional fluid, generally to the back of the foot and towards the outside. Use pressure from your fingers to push out the fluid. Blot the fluid away with a tissue. Clean and dry the skin before doing further blister care. The outer layer of dead skin should not be removed. It is important that the blister not be allowed to refill with fluid. Use one of the blister care products in the next section to protect the blister. Occasionally re-check the blister and drain it again if it has refilled with fluid.

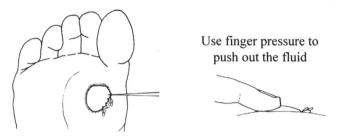

Use finger pressure to push out the fluid

Puncturing a blister with a needle

A better than normal method to drain blisters is to use standard nail clippers or small pointed scissors and clip a hole at the edge at the most dependent spot and also at 180-degrees from there. This lets both gravity and capillary action, along with muscular movement to fully empty the blister. The clippers make a "V" notch, rather than a simple hole. Dan Simpson, DVM, reports, "I have never had a complication from this method and the clippers are easier to manipulate than scissors due to the shorter distance from your hand to the business end. The clipper also functions as a built in depth gauge, preventing too deep an incision."

There is a way to help blisters drain better when hiking or running is required. Ray Zirblis picked this a tip on draining blisters while running the six-day Marathon des Sables in Morocco. Tom Ripley taught him how to drain blisters during stage races or multi-days where a runner will need to keep running. At the end of the days run or other effort, having found blisters and deciding to drain them, one does so, but adds another step. Sterilize a needle and a few inches of thread with alcohol, then thread the needle, and run the needle and thread through one side of the blister and out the other, leaving the thread in place with a 1/4 to 1/2 an inch tail hanging on either end. The thread acts as a wick to further drain any moisture in the blister while one is running or sleeping. Ray reports, "I found that my blisters dried more thoroughly overnight than normal for me, and the inside was much less raw and less sensitive than usual."

Do not drain a blister when it is blood-filled. To do so creates the risk of a serious infection as bacteria is easily introduced into the dermis layer of skin and into the blood system. Pad around the blister with moleskin or adhesive felt.

Do not drain the blister if the fluid inside appears to be either cloudy or hazy. Normal blister fluid is clear and the change indicates that an infection has set in. The fluid needs to be drained, an antibiotic ointment applied, and a protective covering applied. Recheck the blister three times a day for signs of the infection returning. At that time, apply a new coating of antibiotic ointment and change the dressing. Early treatment can keep the infection from becoming more serious.

If the blister has ruptured, the degree of repair depends on the condition of the blister's outer covering. Clean around the blister as described below and apply one of the blister care methods described in the next section can treat a ruptured blister—if the skin is generally intact.

If the outer layer of skin is torn off or only a flap of skin is left, carefully cut off the loose skin, clean the area and cover the new skin with one of the blister care methods described in the next section. Valerie Doyle uses a hair dryer on the blister when the outer layer of skin has been removed or torn off. She has found the low heat and drying action speeds the healing process.

Preventing Infection

The use of soap and water, an antibiotic ointment, Betadine, or hydrogen peroxide for open blisters is important to avoid infection. While you may not use these on an open blister while in the middle of a run or the middle of the day while backpacking, at the end of the event or day, take the necessary time to properly treat the open skin. Check your local drug store for a broad-spectrum antibiotic ointment like Neosporin or Polysporin that provides protection against both gram-positive and gram-negative pathogens. Brave Soldier Wound Healing Ointment is an excellent all-purpose salve to have on hand for blister care.

Blisters should be rechecked daily for signs of infection. An infected blister may be both seen and felt. An infection will be indicated by any of the following: redness, swelling, red streaks up the limb, pain, fever, and pus. The blister must be treated as a wound. It must be frequently cleaned and an antibiotic ointment applied. Frequent warm water or Epsom Salt soaks can also help the healing process. Stay off the foot as much as possible and elevate it above the level of your heart. If the infection does not seem to subside over 24 to 48 hours, see a doctor.

Products

Adhesive Felt   Adhesive felt is available in rolls in 1/8″ and 1/4″ thicknesses. This pink felt is extra thick, and compared to moleskin, provides extra cushioning and a stronger adhesive base. Check with your local drug store, medical supply store, or podiatrist for its availability. Hapad Inc. is a mail-order source for adhesive surgical felt made from a rayon and wool blend in a roll 1/4″ thick by 6″ by 7.5 feet. For more information contact Hapad Inc., PO Box 6, 5301 Enterprise Blvd., Bethel Park, PA 15102; (800) 544-2723; www.hapad.com.

Brave Soldier Wound Healing Ointment   This ointment was made for athletes and is popular among bicyclists. Developed by a dermatologist as an effective treatment to keep abrasion wounds moist and protected, Brave Soldier helps heal blisters, road rash, minor cuts and burns. Made with tea tree oil as a natural antiseptic, aloe gel for its natural healing properties, jojoba oil as a natural moisturizer, Vitamin E to rebuild collagen and skin tissue, shark liver oil to reduce scarring, and comfrey to stimulate skin cell growth and wound resurfacing. For more information contact Brave Soldier, 8330 Beverly Blvd., Los Angeles, CA 90048; (888) 711-BRAV; www.bravesoldier.com.

Moleskin   Moleskin is a soft, cotton padding which protects skin surfaces against friction and has an adhesive backing which adheres to the skin. Dr. Scholl's makes Moleskin Plus from thin cotton flannel padding and Moleskin Foam from soft latex foam. Moleskin is available in most drug stores, in a variety of sizes and can be cut to the size needed. Hapad Inc. is a mail order source for moleskin in a roll 1/8″ thick by 6″ by 7.5 feet. Moleskin should not be applied directly over a blister because it can tear any loose blister skin when removed.

Spenco Pressure Pads   Spenco Pressure Pads are made from closed-cell polyethylene foam which is soft, flexible and thin. It is available in a six-pack of 3″ by 5″ sheets with two pre-cut pads with ovals and circles and two uncut pads to be used over hot spots and blisters. For more information contact Spenco Medical Corporation, PO Box 2501, Waco, TX 76702-2501; (800) 877-3626; www.spenco.com.

Advanced Blister Care

Even though the time-honored blister care products are still used by many, there are more efficient products to both prevent blisters and promote healing.

The chapter *Taping for Blisters* contains much information that can be used as treatments for blisters. See the sections *Taping Basics* on page 91, *Duct Tape Techniques* on page 94, and *Suzi's Taping Techniques* on page 97 for a complete description on how to use taping as a treatment. By following the methods described, tape can be applied over a blister, whether the blister roof is intact or not. Tape can also be applied over Spenco 2nd Skin or other blister care products mentioned below.

Tincture of benzoin applied to the area around a hot spot or blister will help blister products or tapes stick to the skin more effectively. Avoid getting tincture into a ruptured blister or other broken skin. After the tincture has dried, apply one of the blister care products below. Be sure to apply a light coating of powder or lubricant to counteract the still exposed tincture of benzoin to prevent socks or contaminants from sticking to the skin. Be forewarned that forgetting this step when using tincture of benzoin on the toes may result in blisters from two toes being stuck together.

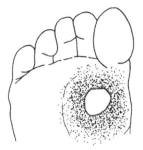 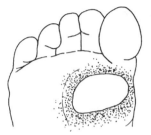

Tincture of benzion applied   Blister product placed over
around blister   blister

When using any of the products listed below on your blisters, be sure to occasionally check them. They may peel off, shift their position, or ball up under the stresses of hiking and running. When doing hills, the constant uphill and downhill movements of the feet combined with the pressures of the running body or the weight of a backpack may compromise their integrity. If you sense a change in how they feel, stop and check it out.

Products

Blister Relief   Blister Relief (formerly Compeed) is a blister cushion made with an elastic polyurethane film over a moisture absorbing and adhering layer, both covered with protective silicone papers that are removed for use. Functioning like a second layer of skin, Blister Relief cushions the area, virtually eliminating blister pain, while protecting it from further damage caused by friction. Tapered edges help adherence to the skin without rolling. It is meant to be used without being cut and can be worn for several days. For larger blisters, put two pieces side-by-side. Be careful not to wrinkle the edges of the pads.

Blister Relief's hydrocolloid construction creates optimum conditions for rapid healing while embedded cellulose particles absorb excess fluid and perspiration from the wound surfaces.

Additionally, bacteria are sealed out, reducing the risk of infection. These pads can be left on until they come off on their own.

Long-distance hiker and ultrarunner Brick Robbins uses tincture of benzoin around his blisters and then applies a Blister Relief pad. The pad usually will stay on for three to five days before falling off. After dealing with massive blisters, Steve Benjamin learned to use a Blister Relief pad placed over each spot prone to blistering, overlapping them where necessary. He then puts tape over the Blister Relief pads to hold them in place. Using five pads per foot, he has eliminated his blister problem. This type of trial can be done with any blister prevention products. Scott Weber wraps the strips around his little toes to protect their blister-prone bottoms. Scott also uses Elastikon tape to anchor the pads to his forefeet..

Blister Relief comes in two sizes, a 3/4" by 2 1/4" strip and a 1 5/8" by 2 5/8" oval, which are available in plastic compacts with either four (oval) or five (strips) pieces. Look for Blister Relief at drug, running, and sports stores. Blister Relief can also be ordered through Medco Sports Medicine, see page 273.

New-Skin Liquid Bandage   New-Skin Liquid Bandage comes in either an antiseptic spray or liquid that is useful as a skin protectant or toughener to prevent hot spots and blisters. It dries rapidly to form a tough protective cover that is antiseptic, flexible, and waterproof, while letting the skin breathe. The one-ounce size is small and convenient. Clean the skin, spray or coat, and let dry. A second coating may be added for additional protection. Keep toes bent when applying and drying. There is no residue or stickiness. Do not apply to infected or draining sites. It is strong smelling stuff, so use with good ventilation and avoid breathing too deeply. Its main ingredients are pyroxylin solution, acetone ACS, oil of cloves, and 8-hydroxyquinoline. Look for New-Skin at drug stores. For more information contact Medtech Laboratories Inc. PO Box 1683, Jackson, WY 83001; (800) 443-4908.

Mueller's More Skin   Mueller's More Skin pads have the feel and consistency of human skin, removing friction between two moving surfaces. More Skin is available in 3" circles, 1" circles and squares, and 3" squares. Available only through wholesale purchase. For more information contact Mueller Sports Medicine, Inc., One Quench Drive, Prairie du Sac, WI 53578; (800) 356-9522; www.muellersportsmed.com; sells only through distributors.

Spenco 2nd Skin Dressings   2nd Skin Dressings are a unique skin-like hydrogel pad that can be applied directly over closed or open blisters. The pads help reduce friction and the discomfort of blisters. They can also be used over abrasions, cuts, or similar wounds. Use one or more pads to cover the blister area. Remove the cellophane layer on one side of the pad, apply that gel side to the blister, and then remove the cellophane from the other side. The pads do not stick to the skin, requiring tape to hold them on the skin. They should be kept moist and changed daily. Cover the 2nd Skin pads with either Spenco Adhesive Knit, one of the tapes mentioned, moleskin, or a self-adhering wrap. These pads are available in a variety of sizes: 1″ squares, 3″ circles, and 3″ by 6.5″ rectangles. Some sizes are non-sterile while others are sold as sterile Moist Burn Pads. Be sure to keep your packet of pads moist or they will dry out. For more information contact Spenco Medical Corporation, PO Box 2501, Waco, TX 76702-2501; (800) 877-3626; www.spenco.com.

Spenco 2nd Skin Blister Pads   These 2nd Skin Blister Pads are made to be applied directly over blisters. Made with the 2nd Skin hydrocolloid pad bordered with a thin adhesive film, the pads keep blisters from drying out, absorbs moisture and perspiration, and promotes a scab free naturally, healed blister. Pads are 60mm by 45mm in an oval shape. For more information contact Spenco as listed above.

Spenco Adhesive Knit   Use Spenco Adhesive Knit to cover 2nd Skin pads or as a skin protector to prevent blisters. Spenco Adhesive Knit is a highly breathable woven fiber with the ability to stretch and conform and does not sweat or bathe off. It cuts to size, fitting easily around toes and hard to tape areas. Adhesive Knit comes in 3″ by 5″ rectangles in a six-pack. For more information contact Spenco as listed above.

Spyroflex   Spyroflex is an adhesive sterile wound dressing. It consists of a thin two-layered polyurethane membrane that has an adhesive inner side which goes against the skin and an outer layer which is moisture-vapor-permeable and microporous. As an "intelligent" dressing, Syproflex is open-cell constructed for moisture management that helps protect the blister from external moisture and bacteria while speeding the healing process. Moisture from the blister is absorbed by the porous membrane, passes through, and evaporates. The membrane is water resistant, not allowing water to pass through to the blister. The pad, cut to size, is applied directly over the blister and may be left on for up to seven days, yet is easily removed without sticking or tearing. Spyroflex works extremely well on inflamed and infected blisters. For maximum adherence, use as much of the pad as possible on the skin around the blister and cover the pad with Spenco Adhesive Knit or a similar porous tape. If continuing to run or hike, check the pad occasionally to be sure it remains in place.

Spyroflex is available in an Abrasion Dressing Kit with three 4" square pads, a Blister Dressing Kit with five 2" square pads, and a Skin Savers package with eight pads in the two different sizes. All pads may be cut to size. They are applied directly over the blister, are water resistant, and may be removed without sticking. The 2" and 4" square pads are sterile. For more information contact Outdoor Rx, 2104 Regency Drive, Irving, TX 75062; (800) 531-5731; www.outdoorrx.com.

Coban   Carry a roll of 3M's 2" Coban in your blister repair kit. Coban is a self-adherent wrap that can be used around feet, ankles, and heels to hold blister products in place. Its elasticity and flexibility allows movement of the joints. Since it adheres to itself, it contains no adhesive. Because it is elastic, be careful not to apply it too tight and cause constriction. Your pharmacy or medical supply stores typically carry Coban or similar self-adherent wraps. Most are available in 2", 3", and 4" widths.

Extreme Blister Prevention and Care

There are athletes who may choose to use extreme methods to initially prevent blisters or subsequently treat their blisters in order to continue on in a competitive event. These are aggressive methods. A competitive 100-mile, 24-hour, 48-hour, or six-day run may cause a runner to want to try any means to keep running. Likewise, hikers may need to deal aggressively with blisters when in the middle of a multi-day hike. The team participation rule in an adventure-racing event may force a team member to consider treating blisters in an extreme method.

There are several extreme methods for extreme blister prevention and care. Review the following methods to determine whether one may be useful for you in your running and hiking adventures.

The first extreme method simply uses information from the chapter *Taping for Blisters* that can be used as an aggressive treatment for both blister prevention and treatment. See the sections *Taping Basics* on page 91, *Duct Tape Techniques* on page 94, and *Suzi's Taping Techniques* on page 97 for a complete description on how to tape. By following the methods described, tape can be applied over a blister, whether the blister roof is intact or not.

The second extreme method of blister prevention uses tincture of benzoin, or a similar benzoin based product, and silicone cream. Marv Skagerberg still likes his benzoin and silicone cream combination that worked for him for the last 78 of 86 days of the 1985 cross-country Trans America race. Averaging 43 miles per day through 12 states, Marv did not get a single blister with this method.

- Clean the feet thoroughly and dry completely.
- Coat the feet, heels, soles, and toes with tincture of benzoin.
- Let the feet dry for three minutes, keeping the toes spread. The feet will still be quite sticky.
- Apply a silicone cream. He uses Avon's Silicone Glove that comes in a 1.5-ounce tube and is available through your Avon sales representative.
- Put on a lightweight double-layer sock.
- Reapply the cream every four to six hours and change socks at the same time.

Ultrarunner and former Appalachian Trail record holder David Horton recommends using zinc oxide on blisters when you have an overnight stop or a rest period for the zinc oxide to do its magic. He remembers using the zinc oxide method on blisters when running the Trans-America (across the United States). He advises, "Take a needle and drain the blister, then using the same hole inject zinc oxide back into the blister until it is full of zinc. Put a Band-Aid over that. Many times we would do that in the Trans-Am and the next day the blister would nearly be dried up. It is still the best thing I have seen to do to a blister." David made this blister fix one time on ultrarunner Dusan Marjele, the eventual Trans-Am winner, and he came back several more times because it was so effective.

Bill Trolan, MD, uses C & M Pharmacal's Hydropel Protective Silicone Ointment over Cramer's Tuf-Skin in the same manner as Marvin described above. He recommends reapplying Tuf-Skin, or similar benzoin product, and cream at every sock change.

Dr. Trolan has participated in several Raid Gauloises and served as a medical consultant to adventure racing teams in the Eco-Challenge as well as to Naval Special Warfare. He wrote the *Blister Fighter Guide*,[24] which is included in the Blister Fighter Medical Kit available through Outdoor Research. He describes two more extreme methods of treating blisters, warning that they are "... not for the faint of heart." This treatment method has helped many adventure racers finish their events. The methods are *not* to be used if the blister is infected. After the blister is opened and drained thoroughly and the feet are dried, use one of the following methods to seal down the blister roof.

> *Please note that the following technique with tincture of benzoin can lead to infections and should ONLY be done if you accept the possible consequences.*

- Use a syringe, without a needle, to inject tincture of benzoin directly into the blister. Immediately apply pressure across the top of the blister to evenly seal down the blister's outer layer to the underlying skin. This also pushes out any extra

benzoin. Be forewarned that injecting the benzoin is momen-
tarily painful. Dr. Trolan rates it as an eight on a one to ten
pain scale where "... childbirth and kidney stones are a ten
and a paper cut is a one."

• Use New-Skin Liquid Bandage, instead of benzoin, injected
into the blister. This does not seal the blister either as well or
as long as benzoin but is less painful. He rates it as a five or
six on the pain scale. See page 175 for information on New-
Skin Liquid Bandage.

At the 1996 Western States 100-Mile Endurance Run Teresa
Krall found out the hard way how painful tincture in a blister can
be. The cotton ball used to apply the tincture was dropped into the
dirt and one of her crew mistakenly decided to pour the tincture
directly onto her blistered heel. As Brick Robbins, her pacer, recalls, "The tincture of benzoin was poured before I could object,
followed by a blood curdling scream. After a while (it seemed
like forever), Teresa quit screaming." Teresa recalls the blister
being about half-dollar size and the pain being intense. She would
not do it again unless it was the only method left to let her run, but
would try Blister Relief first. George Freelen, a former Army
Ranger, recalls when he was in the Army he used the tincture to
seal blisters. He vividly remembers, "It hurts like hell, but only
for 15 to 20 seconds." This method is no longer taught or accepted in the Army. The choice is yours. It works to seal the
blister's roof to the inner skin so running and hiking can continue.
But there is definitely pain and always the risk of infection and
there are other methods.

After sealing the blister, Dr. Trolan gives several options.
Apply a coating of tincture of benzoin to help the tape or moleskin
better adhere to the skin. Or you may apply Instant Krazy Glue
over the blister. This layer provides an extra layer of protection
and helps your tape covering better adhere to the skin. Do not use
Krazy Glue in the blister.

For severe cases, Dr. Trolan has used the tincture of benzoin
injection, followed by a coating of tincture of benzoin on top of
the blister, followed by a coating of New-Skin Liquid Bandage,

followed by a layer of Krazy Glue, and finally followed by tape or moleskin. He recommends using an emery board or fine nail file to smooth any rough spots on the blister coating before applying tape or moleskin.

When using tape or moleskin over a blister, apply it as smoothly as possible. Use finger pressure to smooth it evenly across the blister and then repeat the smoothing process several more times after the initial application. Remember to cut the tape or moleskin large enough to extend well beyond the edges of the blister. The most common failure in using tape or moleskin is not allowing enough necessary for good adherence. The larger the blister, the more the tape or moleskin should extend past its edges.

When using moleskin over blisters, he recommends using a razor to shave the moleskin, after it is applied, to remove its tiny fibers. The fibers can later catch on socks, which exerts pull against the blister.

Dr. Trolan suggests caution in using the two extreme methods described above. Possible permanent damage to the skin surfaces is possible. Use these methods only if you are willing to accept the possible consequences.

Using Syringes and Needles

While you may see medical aid station people using syringes with needles to draw out the blister fluid and then to inject the tincture, an explanation is necessary. Syringes with needles must be sterile in order to prevent infection. There is no safe way to dispose of the syringes and needles, or "sharps" as they are called in the medical profession, except in a sharps container. In the outdoors this presents a problem. Syringes and needles should never be used on more than one person.

In this day of hepatitis, HIV, and AIDS, we need to practice universal precautions—in this case gloves and hand washing before each person being worked on. An open blister must be treated as an open wound and the blister's fluid must be treated as a bodily fluid. Additionally, there are two more concerns. With a syringe you might inject more tincture than is necessary to get a good seal or not enough to cover all inner surfaces. By making several small puncture holes in the blister, and using a syringe without a needle, excess tincture can be pushed out when pressure is applied to the roof of the blister. A good seal is then ensured.

Beyond Blisters

There may be times when blisters develop and even with treatment, due to continued running or hiking, additional care is needed. Several things may happen. The skin may slough off and ball up in the sock, leaving raw exposed skin. The skin may stay in place, but fall off when the sock is removed. The raw skin may bleed. When blisters have developed to this point, a choice will have to be made. Continuing to run or hike may lead to infection. Ideally, stay off the feet as much as possible. If you must continue, treat the problem and recheck the dressing frequently.

Sterile wound dressing products will help the healing process. These dressings are typically available only through medical supply stores but may also be ordered through Medco Sports Medicine (see page 273).

- Bristol-Meyers Squibb's DuoDERM and DuoDERM Extra Thin (4″ x 4″ and 8″ x 8″)
- Cramer Products' Nova Derm (4″ x 4″ and 3″ x 6″ glycerine gel formula)
- Mueller Sports Medicine's Dermal Pads (4″ x 4″ closed-cell elastomer)
- Spenco's 2nd Skin Moist Burn Pads (1.5″ x 2″, 2″ x 3″, and 3″ x 4″ thin gel sheets)
- Spyroflex's 2″ and 4″ square pads

Use these products over the blister or raw skin and leave them on as the healing process begins from the inside. The non-adhesive dressings require a Coban or gauze wrap to hold them in place. One of these carried on a multi-day hike could easily save one's feet. Race directors should consider having several in their first-aid kit.

Fixing Blisters, Their Way or Your Way

Running the Marathon des Sables is unlike any other marathon or ultramarathon. The six-day, self-supported race in the Moroccan desert, has 150-miles of sand, sand, and more sand. Cathy Tibbetts, a many time Marathon des Sables finisher, calls it a blisterfest, "Even people who never get blisters get them." While the medical care is adequate and very good, it is not everyone's first choice of blister care. Cathy reports the usual procedure is to lance the blisters, cut the skin off, apply tincture of benzoin, and then apply Blister Relief. While this is not my first choice of treatment, it does work. Runners report a low incident of infection despite the high level of open blisters. Remember that a lack of preparedness on your part means you will be treated as the medical team has been taught.

Dr. Trolan stresses the importance of understanding how your feet change when you add things to them. Adding moleskin and gauze to your foot changes the way your foot fits inside your shoe or boot. The extra thickness of the blister patch changes pressures and angles of the foot inside the shoe. This in turn changes the shoe from its usually "broken-in" fit to that of a "mismatch." New pressure points develop, turning first into new hot spots and then into blisters. The biomechanics of the foot and ankle and leg are altered and the gait changes. Additional problems are likely to develop. Dr. Trolan recommends using as little and as thin a blister patch as possible.

This becomes most important when participating in an event where you do not have control over the blister treatments and how they are applied. Participate in a 100-mile trail event or an Eco-Challenge and you will find medical aid stations manned by podiatrists, podiatry students, nurses, emergency medical technicians, and an assortment of individuals with various medical skills. These individuals will treat your blisters according to what they know and what materials they have available to them. How they treat your blisters may not be how you would like them treated. Most aid stations are stocked with moleskin, Vaseline, and gauze. They may or may not have 2nd Skin, alcohol wipes, and tincture of benzoin. If you want your feet treated with Blister Relief, 2nd Skin or another product, you will have to carry a few pieces of these in your fanny pack. If you want a specific powder or lubricant you will need to carry these in a small container.

Do not hesitate to give medical personnel at these aid stations instruction on how you would like your feet patched. I remember the bulky gauze patch put on the bottom of my right foot in 1986 during the final stages of my first Western States 100-Mile Endurance Run. While it was a good patch job, it simply did not fit right and turned me from a runner into a walker. Be aware of how they are treating your feet. If you prefer a specific method of blister patching, you need to tell them, and be prepared to describe it to them.

27

Sprains and Strains, Fractures and Dislocations

Ankle sprains and strains are common occurrences—some even with resulting fractures. Bones may be broken from falls and twisting motions, and stress fractures may occur as we push ourselves too fast and too soon. A sudden fall with its resulting wrong landing can result in a dislocated ankle or toe. The cause may be rocks or tree roots hidden in leaves or grasses, trail running at night, or twisting motions coming off a curb. Stress fractures are also common among athletes.

Sprains and Strains

Ankles are frequently sprained or strained. A sprain is a stretching or tearing injury to the ligaments that stabilize bones together at a joint. You may experience sudden pain or hear a pop. If you cannot walk after a few minutes of rest or if you heard the infamous "pop," you can be fairly certain you have a sprain. After a sprain the fibrous joint capsule swells and becomes inflamed, discolored, and painful. An x-ray is in order. Delayed treatments for sprains or strains increases the risk of swelling and further injury. One ankle sprain will make one more susceptible
to repeated sprains.

The most common ankle sprain is an "inversion" sprain where the foot rolls to the outside and the ankle turns out. The injured area is the lateral ligament just below the ankle joint on the outside of the foot. An "eversion" sprain where the ankle is turned inward and the medial ligament is injured is less common. In a serious sprain both the lateral and medial ligaments can be injured. An X-ray will reveal whether there is a bone fracture that would require immobilization of the joint.

A strain is the overstretching of a muscle, tendon, or ligament—but without the significant tearing common to a sprain. There may be bleeding into the muscle area that can cause swelling, pain, stiffness, and muscle spasm followed by a bruise.

There are ways to minimize ankle sprains. Always be aware of how your feet land. If you sense your foot starting to roll over, quickly transfer your weight to your other foot. When on the trail, be attentive to changes in the terrain, especially on downhills and in the late afternoon and evenings when shadows change to darkness. On the road, be aware of curbs, manholes and grates, and the slanted, concave surface roadway. On grassy areas, watch for hidden holes and roots. Any of these can trip you up and throw you off balance. Additionally, when tired you are more susceptible to making wrong moves and being slower to respond to sudden terrain changes.

With a severe sprain there is the possibility of a related fracture. If there is a great deal of pain and swelling, and you are unable to bear weight on the foot, a emergency room visit and an x-ray are in order.

Treatments

The initial treatment for a sprain or strain includes the classic RICE treatment, where R = rest, I = ice, C = compression, and E = elevation. Ice your injury within 30-minutes if possible. The first 24 hours are the most critical for beginning treatment. It may take six to eight weeks for an ankle to fully heal. Severe ankle sprains can require a cast for complete immobilization.

Early treatment within the first 24-hours decreases swelling and lessens the risk of additional injury. Initial rest of the foot is also important. A lightly wrapped Ace wrap will provide compression to help keep swelling down while providing support. Apply the Ace wrap from the forefoot towards the ankle. Do not wear the Ace wrap at night. Apply ice for 20 minutes at a time at least four times daily.

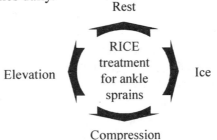

The chapter *Cold & Heat Therapy* on page 257 gives more information on making the most of icing techniques. The injured area should be elevated above the level of the heart as much as possible during the first 48 hours. This keeps blood away from the injured area and reduces pain and swelling. In bed at night, elevate the foot on a pillow. The treatment goal is to return the ankle to normal motion and to be weight bearing as soon as possible. The combination of rest, icing, compression, and elevation, especially in the initial first few days, will help the healing process and decrease the pain and swelling. A mild sprain can take a week to ten days to heal, a serious sprain as long as six to eight weeks.

The use of anti-inflammatory medications is usually warranted. Non-steroidal anti-inflammatory drugs, commonly called NSAIDS, are used to control pain and swelling after an injury. The most common NSAIDS are aspirin, ibuprofen and naproxen sodium (Aleve). These pain relievers should be taken according to their instructions and usually with food. Be care if you continue training because the NSAIDS block pain signals that would warn you of further injury.

Depending on the severity of the injury, you might be able to walk on it. With minimal pain and swelling, self-treatment at home can usually be done. If the pain is severe with a large degree of swelling and there is discoloration of the injured area, prompt medical attention is mandatory.

There are two schools of thought on how soon to start running, exercising, or weight-bear on a twisted injured ankle. The one says to get out on it as soon as possible and let pain be your guide. If the ankle is stiff and sore when you first start, keep going and see if it loosens up. If the pain increases you should call it a day, go home and ice. If it doesn't get worse or feels better you are probably OK. The other says to work through the healing process at the ankle's speed. You must choose your course based on available information.

Certified Athletic Trainer, Jay Hodde, MS, ATC/L, points out that, "Running with a severe sprain can cause more problems than just re-injuring it. Several things may happen.

- Your gait will change as you guard the injury. Because your body is not used to these changes, overuse injuries may occur in other areas of the body.
- The severity of the sprain may increase, prolonging recovery.
- The ankle joint may develop the tendency to partially dislocate (subluxation). This is more common if the sprain is severe. Usually, there is some minor "slipping" of bone surfaces that can cause problems if the joint mechanics are thrown off by the sprain. Bruising of the bone surfaces can occur and can lead to complications later in life, such as an increased risk of arthritis."

When you can start to bear weight on the ankle, start with easy walking and slowly build back to the routine you had before the injury. Wear an ankle support if you cannot bear your full weight on the ankle. Even a little bit a few times a day will aid on the road to recovery. Ice as necessary after each exercise period. Following a few of the strengthening exercises described below will also help gain back ankle strength and normal motion.

Ankle supports are an important part of treating an ankle sprain or strain. The support will allow you to be up and about faster and will provide comfort as the ankle continues healing. There are many types to choose from. The section *Ankle Supports* on page 191 describes an assortment or available supports.

Heat increases blood flow to an injured area, which makes swelling worse. For this reason, the use of heat is not recommended for at least a week after an injury. Moist heat can be applied by using a moist heating pad, a warm towel, or a warm bath. Dry heat can be applied by using a heating pad for 20 minutes at a time.

Since ligaments and tendons do not have their own direct blood supply, their healing is slow. Karl King found that the nutritional supplements of one gram Glycine, one gram Lysine, one-half gram buffered Vitamin C, and one Aleve tablet is helpful in the healing process. Take this combination at breakfast and at bedtime. The supplements provide the major building blocks for connective tissue while the Aleve is an anti-inflammatory.

Two dietary supplements—glucosamine sulfate and chondroitin sulfate have been found to reduce joint pain. Glucosamine sulfate is a natural substance that helps build cartilage, the cushion at the ends of our bones, and maintain joint fluid thickness and elasticity. Chondroitin sulfate, also a natural substance, helps lubricate joints and gives tendons and ligaments their elasticity. Initial studies have found these over-the-counter supplements helpful in stimulating cartilage to grow and inhibiting the enzymes that break down cartilage. Many athletes have added this combination to their daily vitamin and supplement intake as a "must have." Drug stores, pharmacies, and health food stores typically offer these two supplements, typically in one capsule, in an assortment of supplement formulas by different companies. Give these supplements time to work, often a month or more.

Strengthening Exercises

Strengthening exercises for the foot and ankle can help prevent injuries in the first place and will help in recovery from an injury. Balancing exercises are good to help strengthen the ankles. Stop any weight-bearing exercises if you experience pain.

- Sit in a chair and write the alphabet with your toes to simulates ankle motion in all directions.
- Move the ankle up and down in a pumping motion to helps decrease swelling.

- Rotate your feet up to 50 repetitions in each direction. Do four to five sets every other day.
- Strengthen your ankles by balancing with one foot flat on the ground and the other leg bent back at the knee, as if you were in the normal support phase of a running stride. Start at 30 seconds at a time and practice until you can hold your balance for several minutes. When you have mastered this step, close your eyes and do the same thing. Without eye feedback, it is harder to maintain your balance. Repeatedly losing your balance and then recovering gradually strengthens the ankles even more. Mike Bate eliminated ankle problems by doing this one simple exercise. This exercise with your eyes closed works to train your to quickly react to changes as your nerve endings detect a twist or turn when the foot hits the ground.
- Stand on one leg and slowly raise all the way up onto your toes and then slowly lower your heel to a flat foot. Balance yourself as necessary. Start with 25 repetitions and work up to 50 daily.
- Stand with your forefeet on a raised surface, a few inches is fine, and raise up onto your toes and then back down again. Hold each, at the top and at the bottom, for 10-15 seconds. Repeat until both calf's are fatigued.
- Isometric exercises with the feet pushing against each other helps strengthen muscles without joint movement. Push down with the foot on top while pulling up with the foot on the bottom. Then reverse feet. You can also put your feet bottom-to-bottom, first pushing the big toes against each other and then the small toes against each other. Hold the motions for six to ten seconds and repeat several times a day.

Matt Mahoney, one of the proponents of barefoot running and running without socks, feels the most important ankle muscle is the calf. Matt says, "This is what you use to take the weight off your heel and shift to the ball of your foot when your ankle starts to twist." He recommends the following calf exercises, emphasizing "You will know you're doing these exercises right if your calves are sore for several days afterwards."

- Running backwards.
- Running barefoot in sand.
- Stair climbing on real stairs, both up and down. Land on the ball of your foot as you descend.
- Calf raises on a step, with weights, standing for the gastrocnemius and sitting for the soleus. I use machines for these. The standing calf raises are done one foot at a time on a step with a weighted belt. (I use 200 lbs x 10 reps). The sitting raises are done on a machine with weight resting on a padded bar across the top of the legs.

Ankle Supports

Weak ankles can be a problem, particularly on trails. After turning or spraining an ankle, an ankle support will provide the support and protection necessary for light training. Weak ankles can also benefit from an ankle support. Adhesive taping of the ankle can be helpful, however, for it to be effective someone who is experienced must do the taping. While taping restricts extreme motion, the tape loses strength as it moves with the skin. Forty percent of its strength can be lost within 20 minutes.

Ankle supports are typically made from a compression type sock. Some offer a figure-8 style stretch wrap which gives additional strength and support. Since the supports vary in fit and material, experiment wearing the support against the skin or over a sock to find the best fit on your foot. All the ankle supports listed below are compact in size and fit easily into a fannypack or backpack. If you are prone to ankle injuries, consider carrying one as a preventative measure.

Products

AnkleWrap - U-Wrap   The AnkleWrap is a convenient wrap for the ankle that is different than the typical ACE wrap. Made from an open-celled, elastomeric, non-latex foam, the wrap that breathes to wick away perspiration, stays put with superior sticking power, and is fully adjustable. At 10 feet long by 1 1/2 inches wide, it is long enough to make a complete figure-8 wrap with three heel locks. The PrattStrap is a similar wrap made for Patella Tendonitis and ITB syndrome. For more information contact fabrifoam Products, 900 Springdale Drive, Exton, PA 19341; (800) 577-1077; www.fabrifoam.com.

Cho-Pat Ankle Support   The Cho-Pat Ankle Support provides compression to the ankle with a removable Velcro fastener which wraps in a figure-8 around the ankle giving additional compression at specific locations of the ankle while providing stabilization. The support is made of neoprene. The unisex sizes are based on instep circumference. For more information contact Cho-Pat, Inc. PO Box 293, Hainesport, NJ 08036; (800) 221-1601; www.cho-pat.com.

Cropper Medical Bio Skin   Cropper Medical makes Bio Skin, a compression support material. Bio Skin is made up of a hypo-allergenic Lycra knit outer layer, a SmartSkin membrane that absorbs moisture and wicks it from the skin, a Lycra knit/fleece inner layer, and a SkinLok layer against the skin. Bio Skin stretches with the body's movement while giving compression without bunching and binding, and does not constrict the joints. The SmartSkin membrane provides higher levels of moisture vapor transmission as the activity produces more perspiration and heat. The three designs include a standard pull on ankle skin, a figure-8 ankle skin, and a visco ankle skin with a figure-8 wrap that includes visco polymer inserts around malleolus ankle bones. The Bio Skin material will not tear even if cut into. Cropper Medical also makes models for knee problems or injuries, including hinged braces for athletes needing knee support. For more information contact Cropper Medical, 240 East Hersey Street, Suite 2, Ashland, OR 97520; (800) 541-2455.

Kallassy Ankle Support   The Kallassy Ankle Support is a proven design for rehabilitation of severe ankle sprains. The support is made of nylon-lined neoprene that provides warmth and compression. A strap that wraps around the ankle provides stability first and secondly by a non-stretch lateral strapping system that helps prevent inversion motions of the ankle. If you are prone to turned ankles, this support is one of the most stabilizing ankle supports offered. A lace-up version is offered but it would not be as comfortable for running and hiking. The Rebound Orthopedic Supports Division of Tecnol sells the Kallassy. For more information contact Tecnol Consumer Products, 6625 Industrial Park Boulevard, Fort Worth, TX 76180; (800) 832-3182. Also available from Medco Sports Medicine (see page 273).

Perform 8 Lateral Ankle Stabilizer   The Perform 8 provides excellent external stabilization of the ankle's lateral (outer) ligaments, similar to ankle taping. While a lightweight elastic compression sock provides support to soft tissue, an elastic figure-8 configuration strap wraps around the foot. Pads protects and relieve pressure on the Achilles tendon. This support is excellent for athletes prone to chronic ankle sprains. For more information contact Brown Medical Industries, 1300 Lundberg Drive West, Spirit Lake, IA 51360; (800) 843-4395; www.brownmed.com.

TakeOff Ankle Protec Wrap   The Protec ankle wrap uses the fabrifoam material to make a lightweight and thin, slip resistant, breathable wrap with a moisture transfer system. This one size fits most adults wrap provides adjustable compression without bulkiness and will fit inside a shoe. For more information contact Smith+Nephew Inc., One Quality Drive, PO Box 1005, Germantown, WI 53022; (800) 558-8633.

Stromgren Ankle Support   Stromgren Supports makes a good ankle support for general use. Their double strap model offers a unique sock style support with two elastic straps that wrap around the ankle to provide the benefit of taped ankle support without the tape. This product fits fairly loose and has folded-over sewn edges at the forefoot and the heel cutout that might be irritating on extended hikes or runs. For more information contact Stromgren Supports, PO Box 1230, Hayes, KS 67601; (913) 625-9036.

Other Ankle Supports   Additional ankle supports can usually be found in drug stores and sporting goods stores. Three examples are those made by Cramer, Mueller, and Spenco. Cramer's neoprene ankle support wraps around the ankle. Mueller's

Neoprene Ankle Support is a one-piece support with stretch nylon on each side. The Spenco Fiberflex is an elastic bandage for the ankle made from elastic and transverse nylon fibers. Ace wraps, or similar style elastic wraps are helpful after a sprain, but provide little support against initially turning your ankle.

Fractures

Any bone in the foot can fracture however some are more prone to injury than others. The terms *break* and *fracture* are synonymous— there is a structural break in the continuity of the bone. A fracture may occur from a fall, the twisting motion of an turned ankle, a blow from hitting your foot on a rock or tree root, or simply from a bad foot plant. In the foot the toes are most likely to fracture— usually the first (big toe) and the fifth (small toe). A common foot fracture is the Jones fracture, a fracture of the fifth metatarsal on the outside of the foot. This type of fracture is common with a fall or loss of balance where you put a sudden and undue amount of pressure on the outside of your foot. There are many types of fractures.

- Avulsion – the tearing away of a part of the bone attached to a ligament or tendon
- Butterfly – a bone fragment shaped like a butterfly and part of a comminuted fracture
- Complete – the bone is completely broken through
- Comminuted – more than two fragments, may be splintered
- Displaced – bone fragments are moved away from each other
- Impacted – fragments are compressed by force into each other or adjacent bone
- Incomplete – the continuity of the bone is destroyed on only one side
- Nondisplaced – the bone pieces are still together in the correct locations/angles
- Segmental – several large fracture in the same bone
- Spiral – the fracture line is spiral in shape

Fractures usually manifest themselves with a great deal of pain and tenderness directly above the fracture site. Where there is soft tissue injury, there will also be discoloration of the skin above the fracture. Fractures that are ignored can result in a malunion or non-union of the pieces of bone that should have mended correctly together. This could require surgery to correctly align the bone ends.

The Ottowa Ankle Rules[25] are often used by emergency room physicians and sports specialists to determine, before an x-ray, the likelihood of an ankle fracture. The study takes two approaches.

- Pain in the malleolar (ankle bones) zone and either: 1) inability to bear weight immediately and in the emergency room (four steps), or 2) bone tenderness at the posterior (back) edge of either malleolus.
- Pain in the midfoot zone and either: 1) inability to bear weight immediately and in the emergency room (four steps), or 2) bone tenderness at the navicular (the bone at the top front of the foot at the curve up the ankle) or fifth metatarsal (the midfoot bone on the outside of the foot).

Treatments

Treatment for fractures is the typical combination of rest, ice, immobilization, and elevation. Toe fractures are usually buddy taped and the patient is advised to wear a firm soled shoe, or a wooden orthopedic shoe that restricts flexion of the foot. A fracture of the big toe can warrant a full foot cast. A Jones fracture or any other fracture of the foot or ankle will require a cast and immobilization for between four to six weeks. The rule of thumb with fractures is to immobilize the joint above and the joint below the fracture. You may start out with a non weight-bearing cast, requiring the use of crutches, and later have it changed to a weight-bearing walking cast. Refer to the chapter *Cold & Heat Therapy* on page 257 for more information on making the most of icing techniques.

Stress Fractures

Stress fractures are a common sports injury. Sudden or repetitive stress, usually from overuse without proper conditioning, results in a small crack in the outer shell of the affected bone. Over time, if not treated, this crack will develop into a fracture of the bone. The most common foot bones to stress fracture are the second and third metatarsal bones in the forefoot—between the toes and the ankle. Some doctors will use an x-ray to make the diagnosis. Often a stress fracture does not show on an initial x-ray because the bone's callus formation has not yet taken place at the fracture site. A bone scan, different from an x-ray, is useful for a questionable diagnosis and will usually confirm whether you have a stress fracture. Some hospitals will use an MRI to make the diagnosis. Often there is no recollection of having injured the foot.

Other possible causes of stress fractures include wearing worn out or poor-fitting shoes, ill-fitting insoles, abnormal foot structure or mechanics (arch or pronation problems, or leg-length discrepancies), or tightness and inflexibility. Your medical specialist may recommend additional calcium in your diet and/or bone density testing. Female athletes who have infrequent periods are most at risk for stress fractures.

There is typically pain to the touch, often first felt as a dull ache or soreness at the point of the stress fracture. The pain usually becomes worse as the break grows. Swelling is common. Stress fractures are most common from overuse, over training, or a change in running surfaces—from a softer to a harder surface. Stress fractures are also referred to as "march fractures."

Peter Fish remembers his first stress fracture, the 3rd metatarsal of the right foot, that happened in July of '95. His second fracture may have started as a stress fracture or may have simply been a fracture from the start.

I had had an unpleasant "itchy" sensation on the top of my foot for a month or so (I was ramping up mileage for the Portland Marathon), and during a training run it turned into a sudden sharp pain. I limped home and went to my family doctor the same day. The fracture didn't show on the X-ray yet, but it appeared a couple of weeks later when I consulted my podiatrist. I didn't use the walking boot, but if I had to do a lot of walking I found that a stiff-soled pair of medium high work boots kept my foot from flexing painfully and enabled me to walk almost normally. I didn't run for six weeks, then started off cautiously, this time with the California International Marathon (early December) in mind.

This time my training went quite well, with no protests from the injured foot, and I was able to get up to 40 miles a week with five or six long runs. I ran two races during the month or so before the marathon, one of nine miles and the other of 20k, both at my projected marathon pace. A couple of weeks before the race, the top of my left foot felt sore. My podiatrist thought it was probably a neuroma from too tight laces, as it was rather high up on the instep for a stress fracture. I ran the marathon, in some discomfort, although this didn't seem to get worse during the race, and I managed to attain my Boston qualifier by a couple of minutes with a time of 3:38. Immediately after the race, my foot became extremely painful, and I could hardly walk on it. It was a couple of weeks before I could run at all, and I had to run on the outside of that foot to do it. It didn't seem to be healing at all, so I went back to the podiatrist. An X-ray showed it to be fractured quite badly, nearly all the way through. The reason I could run on it was that the break was near the top of the (third) metatarsal, where there was less flexion. The doctor thought it seemed more like a break due to trauma than a normal stress fracture. During the 9-mile race I had run a couple of months before, I got off the course once and had to jump a ditch to get back. I landed pretty heavily, and it seemed possible that this set up the fracture, which came on later, possibly during the marathon. The regimen was the same as before: no running for six weeks, and as before, I spent a lot of time in the pool, on my bike, and even did some cross-country skiing.

Treatments

After a confirming scan, a sports doctor, orthopedists, or podiatrist will usually recommend at least six weeks off. Follow their advice. To run or exercise heavily on a stress fracture is asking for more problems. Switch to more cushioned shoes and use this recovery time to focus on other non-weight bearing exercises and cross-training: cycling, pool running, swimming, and weight training. Ask your doctor whether you can use a limited-weight bearing exercise machine like a stair climber or elliptical trainer.

An Ace wrap or compression sock will help control swelling. A orthopedic or wooden shoe may be used to splint the foot. Anti-inflammatories are helpful. Elevation of the foot above the level of the heart will help reduce pain and swelling. Ice the area 20-minutes at a time three to four times a day and after any exercise. The *Cold & Heat Therapy* chapter on page 257 gives more information on making the most of icing techniques. Difficult cases may require splinting, casting, or surgery.

Dislocations

A dislocation is a complete displacement of bone from its normal position at a joint's surface, which disrupts the articulation of two or three bones at that junction and alters alignment. The dislocation may be complete, where the joint surfaces are completely separated, or incomplete (subluxation), where the joint is only slightly displaced. The dislocation may be caused by a direct blow or injury, or by a ligament's tearing.

In the foot the most common dislocations are the toes. Any of the toes can be dislocated but the most common are the big toe or the small toe.

The ankle can be dislocated by any combination of fractures of the tibia (the big inner bone of the lower leg) or fibula (the small outer bone of the lower leg) resulting in a displaced talus. Ankle dislocations can be a major lower leg injury with severe consequences if the circulation to the foot are compromised.

Treatments

Dislocated toes are fairly simply to treat. Resetting dislocations is called "reduction." With one hand stabilize the ball of the foot with your thumb on the injured toe. With the other hand exert traction to the toe while pushing down, or upward, depending on the angle of the dislocation with the first thumb. This reduces the dislocation. The toe then needs to be "buddy taped" to the toe or toes next to it for stabilization. A small piece of gauze, cotton, or tissue between the taped toes will prevent skin breakdown if the tape is on for any great length of time. A firm soled shoe will help keep the toe in line and the foot-toe joint stable.

To temporarily correct and stabilize an ankle dislocation and related fracture, an orthopedic trauma surgeon recommends straightening the foot by exerting traction in a straight and steady motion—so that as much as possible it is its natural position and angle to the lower leg. The foot, ankle, and lower leg then need to be stabilized with a splint. Use any available materials to keep the extremity stable. Check the toes frequently for normal skin color and warmth which indicates good circulation. An dislocated ankle needs to be treated by an emergency room physician or orthopedic surgeon as soon as possible.

If either a toe or ankle dislocation is an "open" dislocation, where the bone has come through the skin, extra care must be taken. This open, or complex, dislocation is usually associated with a fracture and the bone may still be outside of the skin or may have pulled back inside. First, clean the wound, then proceed with the reduction. Then, leaving the wound open, apply a sterile dressing, and splint the extermity. Check the end(s) of the extremity farthest from the body to be sure there is adequate circulation, adjusting the extremity as necessary.

28

Heel Problems

The most common cause of heel pain is incorrect movement of the foot during running, hiking, or walking. With every heel strike, pressure up to four times the body's weight is placed on the heel, flattening the heel's fat pads and sending shock and stress to the bones of the foot and the arch. Some of the shock and stress travels on up the leg. As we age, the thickness of the heel's fat pads (and the fat pads under the balls of our feet) decreases and our natural shock absorption is reduced, pressure is increased, and we become more susceptible to injury.

Heel pain may also be caused by heel spurs or plantar fasciitis as the heel bone and attached soft tissues are stressed. This type of heel pain is often the worst in the morning after getting out of bed and putting your feet on the floor—sometimes improving after a few minutes. Any athlete with heel pain should also read the next chapter on *Plantar Fasciitis*. Often heel pain is related to problems with the plantar fasica.

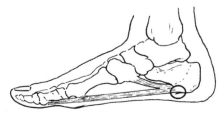

Heel spur at the bottom
of the heel bone

Heel spurs are small points of calcium buildup sticking out and downward from the "calcaneus" heel bone, touching and irritating your plantar fascia. Stresses to the plantar fascia where it inserts into the calcaneus cause heel spurs to develop. A heel spur can usually be seen on an x-ray. A heel bruise or stone bruise is pain felt directly under the calcaneus. This pain is usually tenderness at a small site just forward of the heel's pad on the bottom of the heel.

Treatments

Heel pads and cups may help heel pain caused by heel spurs, plantar fasciitis, calcaneal bursitis, heel neuromas, and nerve entrapment syndromes. Proper conditioning of the feet and gradually working up to longer distances can help minimize heel pain. Resting your feet and using ice is helpful when you first experience pain—20 minutes three to four times a day for several days. The chapter *Cold & Heat Therapy* on page 257 gives more information on making the most of icing techniques. Later, warm soaks can help. If the problem persists, make an appointment with a podiatrist or orthopedist.

One very basic, but important recommendation is to never walk in bare feet until you are pain free—even in the morning getting out of bed. Keep a pair of sandals of shoes at your bedside.

A study by the American Orthopaedic Foot and Ankle Society looked at heel pain related to plantar fasciitis.[26] Dr. Glenn Pfeffer reported chronic heel pain as the most common foot problem with up to 80% caused by proximal plantar fasciitis. The study compared a common polypropylene custom orthotic device, three over-the-counter heel pads, and stretching alone. After comparing the results of five control groups, they found that stretching and over-the-counter heel pads were as effective as stretching and the more costly orthotics. Their recommendation is "... for the initial treatment of heel pain, stretching, and a simple, inexpensive, off-the-counter device is the best way to go." When wearing heel pads, be sure to use them in all your shoes.

The products listed below are quite varied. Some heel cups have a waffle design or special-density bottom material on the bottom of the cup, others have a U-shape cutout at the bottom of the heel. Most heel cups simply cup the heel while others are incorporated into a sock design. The new viscoelastic materials in some heel pads provide excellent cushioning. Heel pads are small and fit easily into a shoe to provide cushioning. Try several to find a design that works best for your pain or injury. Heel cups and pads are small and can easily be carried as a preventive measures if you are prone to heel pain. The Count'R-Force Arch Brace and the PSC wrap are alternatives to heel cups and pads. The Strassburg Sock can be worn at night or while resting to lightly stretch the plantar fascia. Several off-the-counter orthotics are also available.

Heel pain can also be caused by dry and cracked skin at the back and bottom of the heel. This skin is often built up into a callus and the fissures in the skin can be painful. Treat this problem the same as a callus. See the chapter *Corns, Calluses, Bunions, and Bursitis* on page 241 for common treatments.

Stretching Exercises

Stretching can help resolve heel pain. Warm soaks and stretching after extended sitting can also be beneficial.

- Slowly stretch the toes upward towards the head at least three times per day, holding the stretch for at least 15 seconds. Do this stretching in the morning before getting out of bed.
- An easy and effective exercise is to sit on a stool or other surface that permits your legs to dangle and point your toes downward as you draw the alphabet in the air. Repeat three to five times.
- Dr. Les Appel, who designed the Power*step* Insole recommends facing a wall with one foot flat on the floor and the other foot's heel on the floor and toes up on the wall 3-4 inches. Gently move your knee slowly towards the wall until you feel slight stretching on the bottom of your foot and the back of your leg. Hold this position for 30 seconds, repeating five times per foot.

The ProStretch is a popular tool to effectively relieve heel pain by stretching the plantar fascia, while also stretching the Achilles tendon and the gastrocnemius and soleus musculature of the back of the lower leg.

Products

Accommodator Orthotics   AliMed offers several orthotics to provide relief from heel pain and plantar fasciitis. The High-Impact Accommodator offers the benefit of an Impact Plus energy-absorbing poromeric polymer pad in the heel. The new Viscoelastic Accommodator uses a viscoelastic polymer that cradles the heel while providing cushioning and shock absorption. Each offers a shaped longitudinal arch to relieve fatigue while supporting the arch and a mild metatarsal arch to support and reduce unnecessary pressure from the metatarsal heads. For more information contact AliMed Inc.,297 High Street, Dedham, MA 02026-9135; (800) 225-2610; www.alimed.com.

Count'R-Force Arch Brace   Taping of the foot can help but is difficult to do on yourself. The brace is an alternative to taping and is ideal for running and hiking. Designed by Robert Nirschi, MD., an Orthopedic Surgeon/Sports Medicine Specialist, its curved shape allows a wide distribution of the abusive forces causing heel and plantar fasciitis pain. Made to fit either foot, an adult universal or small size will fit most individuals. Two tension straps allow for personal adjustment. For more information contact Medical Sports, Inc., PO Box 7187, Arlington, VA 22207; (800) 783-2240; www.medsports.com.

Cramer Heel Cup   Cramer Products offers a basic heel cup made with Provosane II bonded to soft polyurethane foam. For more information contact Cramer Products Inc. PO Box 1001, Gardner, KS 66030; (800) 255-6621; www.cramersportsmed.com. Available through distributors or from Medco Sports Medicine (see page 273).

Hapad Heel Pads and Cushions   Hapad's Heel Cushions are useful in treating heel pain associated with stone bruises, heel spurs, leg length discrepancies, and Achilles tendinitis. The Horseshoe Heel Pads relieve heel pain and the Medial/ Lateral Heel Wedges help correct misalignment of the heel and ankle. The Comf-Orthotic 3/4-Length Insole is a contoured one-piece arch, metatarsal, and heel cushion which relieves heel spur pain. The coiled, spring-like wool fibers provide firm and resilient support as they mold and shape to the foot. For more information contact Hapad Inc., PO Box 6, 5301 Enterprise Blvd., Bethel Park, PA 15102; (800) 544-2723; www.hapad.com.

Heel Bed 4pf UCO International makes a Heel Bed 4pf, a molded polymer orthotic device for the relief of heel pain secondary to plantar fasciitis. Its molded design cups the heel and has an arch support. These are made in sizes small, medium, and large. This heel bed has to be ordered through a distributor, a podiatrist, or an orthopedist through UCO International, professional reorders only: (800) 541-4030.

Heel Hugger The Heel Hugger is designed to treat heel pain and inflammatory problems of the heel. The neoprene sock design surrounds the foot from the heel to the mid-foot providing support, stabilization, and compression to control edema. Therapeutic Gel pads with Sealed Ice provide additional stabilization and cold therapy on either side of the calcaneus heel bone. The Heel Hugger provides relief from heel spurs, plantar fasciitis, Achilles tendinitis, heel contusions, narrow heels, and rearfoot instability. For more information contact Brown Medical Industries, 1300 Lundberg Drive West, Spirit Lake, IA 51360; (800) 843-4395; www.brownmed.com.

Lynco Biomechanical Orthotic Systems Apex offers the Lynco Biomechanical Orthotic System, a "ready-made" triple-density orthotic system that comes in enough variations to accommodate 90% of foot disorders, including pain from heel spurs and heel pain syndrome. See the chapter *Orthotics* on page 115 for more information about Lynco orthotics. For more information contact Apex Foot Health Industries, Inc., 170 Wesley Street, So. Hackensack, NJ 07606; (800) 526-2739; www.apexfoot.com.

Power*step* Insoles The Power*step* insoles was design by a Dr. Les Appel to provide complete heel and arch support and stability. Its strong heel cradle prevents the foot from pronating (rolling inward) or the arch from flattening—eliminating strain on the plantar fascia. For more information contact Power*step*, PO Box 46744, Cincinnati, OH 46744; (888) 237-3668; www.powerstep.com.

ProStretch This popular tool effectively stretches the plantar fascia, the Achilles tendon, and the calf muscles. The ProStretch builds lower extremity strength, balance, and flexibility benefits in three minutes of use prior to activity, thus reducing the risk of injury. The PT100 is unilateral while the PT200 is bilateral. Both models can also be used for hamstring and anterior tibialis stretching. For more information contact ProStretch at Prism Enterprises, 6952 Fairgrounds Parkway, San Antonio, TX 78238; (800) 535-3629; www.prostretch.com.

PSC - Pronation/Spring Control The PSC stands for Pronation/Spring Control device. It is designed to treat chronic heel pain, heel spur syndrome, plantar fasciitis, and shin splints. This reusable strapping device is made from an open-celled, elastomeric, non-latex foam. It breathes to wick away perspiration, stays put with superior sticking power, and is fully adjustable. It wraps under the arch to provide superior support to the plantar fascia and then around the heel to reduce the force of heel strike and biomechanically move the foot's mid-line to a more neutral position. For more information contact fabrifoam Products, 900 Springdale Drive, Exton, PA 19341; (800) 577-1077; www.fabrifoam.com

Spenco Jam Wrap Support Spenco offers a Polysorb Heel Cup made from molded polyurethane combined with a neoprene ankle wrap—it pulls on like a sock. For more information contact Spenco Medical Corporation, PO Box 2501, Waco, TX 76702-2501; (800) 877-3626; www.spenco.com.

Spur Relief Heel Cup Orthopedic Product Sales makes a Spur Relief Heel Cup with silicone that has a density similar to that of human tissue. For more information contact Orthopedic Product Sales, 975 Old Henderson, Columbus, OH 43220; (800) 992-9999; sells only through distributors.

Strassburg Sock This unique sock is easy to use at night or extended periods of rest. A standard over-the-calf tube sock uses two adjustable straps, one around the calf just below the knee, the other attached to the toe of the sock and passed through a "D" ring on the upper strap. Tension on the toe strap keeps the plantar fascia in a neutral to slightly stretched position, eliminating in the reduction or elimination of pain under the heel during initial weight bearing in the morning. A good alternative to the typical night splint. For more information contact JT Enterprises LLC, PO Box 1253, N. Tonawanda, NY 14120; (800) 452-0631; www.thesock.com.

The Ultimate Heel & Arch Support   Made by footcare specialist, Dr. G. Budak, the Ultimate is made from viscoelastic polymer that molds to the foot, forms a deep heel cup, and follows the contour of the arch, thereby making a custom fit. As a 3/4-length orthotic, it provides relief from plantar fasciitis, heel spur pain, Achilles tendonitis, and arch, knee, and back strain. It also absorbs up to 90% of shock which reduces stress to the heel, foot, leg, and back. For more information contact The Foot Store, 1909 N. Highway 17, Mount Pleasant, SC 29464; (800) 775-3668; www.footstore.com.

Tuli's Heel Cups Tuli's makes different versions of heel cups. The TuliGel Heel Cup offers a double-ribbed waffle design with gel polymer that is soft but strong. Their Tuli's Pro Heel Cup has a double-ribbed waffle design while the Tuli's Cheetah Neoprene Ankle Support incorporates a Tuli's Standard Heel Cup with a neoprene ankle sock-type support. For more information contact Allor Medical, Inc. 109 White Oak Lane #92, Old Bridge, NJ 08857; (800) 444-TULI.

Viscoheel   Viscoheel Heel Cushions are made from a non-compressible, viscoelastic material. They reduce shock to the joints and evenly distributes pressure throughout the cushion. Made to relieve heel pain associated with heel spurs, thinning heel pads, and plantar fasciitis. Three versions are available. For more information contact Bauerfeind USA, Inc., 2100 Barrett Park Drive, Suite 508, Kennesaw, GA 30144; (800) 423-3405; www.bauerfeind.com. Available through distributors or from Medco Sports Medicine (see page 273).

Some runners and hikers may find relief using a basic heel cushion—a simple pad that fits under the heel of the foot. Spenco and Spectrum Sports offer heel cushions. Check your running, backpacking, or drug stores for these and similar products.

29

Plantar Fasciitis

The plantar fascia is a band of connective fibrous tissue that runs from the heel to the ball of the foot, forming the foot's arch. The band aids in support and stabilization of the foot during hiking and running. The arch flattens when standing. As you begin a step the heel lifts up and the plantar fascia tightens to form the curve of the arch and provides a strong push off with the toes. An inflammation of the fascia, called plantar fasciitis, most often occurs with overuse. The stretching and tearing of some of the fibers in the plantar fascia as it inserts into the heel bone causes the inflammation. If you have flat feet or if you over-pronate, the plantar fascia is strained, mainly at the heel. The stresses of impact sports, running, and hiking may flatten, lengthen, and eventually cause small tears in the plantar fascia. Tears near the heel bone may cause a heel spur to develop. Running and hiking hills may further stress the foot.

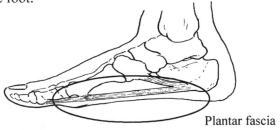

Plantar fascia

Plantar fascia pain is commonly felt in the morning or after long periods of sitting. The first steps at these times causes a sudden strain to the band of tissue. There may be either heel or arch pain. The pain and stiffness is usually centered at the bottom of the heel, but symptoms may radiate into the arch. Although the pain may decrease somewhat with your initial activity, as the day progresses, it may return and be quite painful.

Consult your podiatrist or orthopedist if you are suffering from pain in the arch of your foot or suspect that you have plantar fasciitis. An aggressive multi-disciplined medical approach using medical, biomechanical, and physical therapy treatments can help to return you to action as soon as possible. The Achilles tendon may also be involved, causing pain under the foot as it stretches.

In an interesting article, "Plantar Fasciitis—A New Perspective"[27], Robert Nirschl, MD, makes a case for plantar fasciitis as a painful degenerative plantar tendonitis, not an inflammation problem. His research found no inflammatory cells in injured plantar fascia—meaning anti-inflammatory medications and cortisone will not have curative potential. For plantar tendonitis Dr. Nirschl recommends stretching and strength training to all areas of the leg to restore strength, endurance, and flexibility. Also recommended is the use of a night splint, arch bracing or a soft orthotic, and footwear with good mid-foot flexibility. In extreme cases, surgery may be indicated to remove painful tendonitis tissue. If your plantar fascia pain does not respond to prescribed treatment, consider asking your podiatrist or orthopedist to look into this study.

Treatments

Treatments include rest, moist heat and stretching in the morning or before activity, icing massage after activity, changing insoles or adding an arch support, taping of the foot or an arch brace, foot exercises, and shoe modifications. Replace your worn out shoes and insoles. In extreme cases oral anti-inflammatory medications, cortisone injections, physical therapy, cast immobilization, and even surgery may be necessary. Usually you need either to provide more support to the arch or lessen the amount of over-pronation. An arch support or arch pad can provide pain relief. Motion-control shoes can help if you over-pronate. Ice your heels and the bottom of your foot after exercise. The chapter *Cold & Heat Therapy*, on page 257 gives more information on making the most of icing techniques.

The first thing any doctor or physical therapist should tell you is to stop all impact activities for a period of weeks or months and to always wear shoes. Going barefoot is one of the worst things someone with plantar fasciitis can do. Keep in mind that the tiny tears need to heal and it makes sense to stop the activity that caused them in the first place. You also need to regain flexibility and elasticity in the soleus muscle/sheath to prevent it from happening again. Stretching is the way to do that, but you have to start out slow and easy, i.e., the alphabet in warm bath water. Once you've started to heal, you can move on to the more demanding stretches.

Gary Buffington recommends trying inexpensive orthotic shoe inserts before you have expensive orthotics made. Gary suggests, "Wear them always until you are better—even in your bedroom slippers if you go to the bathroom at night. I think it would be best if you never took a step without them under your foot for a month. Also two Aleve tablets twice a day; and contrast baths of two buckets of water, one at 68 degrees the other 103 degrees. Five minutes in hot, two in cold, five in hot, two in cold, and then five more in the hot for a total of 19 minutes twice a day or more." Following that regiment for one year got Gary through the Boston Marathon.

Like Gary found, orthotics will often help relieve plantar fascia pain. AliMed Rehab and Apex make orthotics for plantar fasciitis. Because self-taping of one's arch is difficult, an arch brace is an easy alternative. Providing support to the arch, an arch brace wraps around the arch in order to provide support and decrease the pull of the plantar fascia on the calcaneus heel bone. The Count'R-Force Arch Brace and the PSC wrap are two wrap-around supports to provide relief from plantar fasciitis pain. The Hapad Longitudinal Metatarsal Arch Pads or 3-Way Heel/Arch/Metatarsal Insoles and the Apex Lynco orthotics may be used to relieve pain.

A lightweight plastic night splint worn to bed can help to stretch the foot, limit contraction of soft tissues at night, and avoid morning stiffness. Night splints help avoid footdrop and accompanying muscle tightening. Night splints are proven as a treatment method of preventing the plantar fascia and Achilles tendon from contracting during the night. Many athletes swear by them. Check with your podiatrist, orthopedist, or medical supply store. Several night splint models are available. The Strassburg Sock is an alternative style night splint which can be worn at night or while resting to lightly stretch the plantar fascia.

Stretching Exercises

Athletes can improve their flexibility and counter muscular imbalances that puts them at a greater risk of injury by following a simple stretching program. The best results may come from a combination of plantar fascia and Achilles tendon stretching in multiple directions.

- Stretching can be easily done by bending the knee with the ankle flexed back towards you and gently pulling your toes back towards your knee. Hold this pull to a count of ten and repeat six to ten times a day. Using a towel around your toes to pull them towards you is an alternative. Do this before getting out of bed in the morning.
- Dr. Les Appel, who designed the Power*step* Insole recommends facing a wall with one foot flat on the floor and the other foot's heel on the floor and toes up on the wall 3-4 inches. Gently move your knee slowly towards the wall until you feel slight stretching on the bottom of your foot and the back of your leg. Curl your toes to raise the arch and transfer your weight to the outside of your foot. Uncurl your toes, hold for 30 seconds and again curl your toes. Hold each position for 30 seconds, repeating five times per position per foot.
- An effective morning calf stretch is to stand facing a wall with your hands on the wall. Extend one foot behind you about 24 inches, while bending the other leg at the knee. Keep the heel of the back foot flat on the floor for a two minutes and keep the knee straight—you will feel the calf muscle stretch. Repeat with the other foot.

- Rolling a tennis ball back and forth under the arch of the foot or simple self-massage across and along the arch can also help. Ice massage can be done using a small frozen juice can rolled under your arch after a run.

The ProStretch is a popular tool to effectively stretch the plantar fascia as well as the Achilles tendon and the gastrocnemius and soleus musculature of the back of the lower leg. Studies have shown that utilization of the ProStretch can more effectively increase ankle dorsiflexion (toe-up motion of the ankle) than by the conventional and commonly used wall stretch technique mentioned above.[28] Its use is recommended as both a preventive measure as well as a treatment technique.

Products

Accommodator Orthotics   AliMed offers several orthotics to provide relief from heel pain and plantar fasciitis. The High-Impact Accommodator offers the benefit of an Impact Plus energy-absorbing poromeric polymer pad in the heel. The new Viscoelastic Accommodator uses a viscoelastic polymer that cradles the heel while providing cushioning and shock absorption. Each offers a shaped longitudinal arch to relieve fatigue while supporting the arch and a mild metatarsal arch to support and reduce unnecessary pressure from the metatarsal heads. For more information contact AliMed Inc., 297 High Street, Dedham, MA 02026-9135; (800) 225-2610; www.alimed.com.

Count'R-Force Arch Brace   Taping of the foot can help but is difficult to do on yourself. The brace is an alternative to taping and is ideal for running and hiking. Designed by Robert Nirschi, MD., an Orthopedic Surgeon/Sports Medicine Specialist, its curved shape allows a wide distribution of the abusive forces causing the heel and plantar fasciitis pain. Made to fit either foot, an adult universal or small size will fit most individuals. Two tension straps allow for personal adjustment. For more information contact Medical Sports, Inc., PO Box 7187, Arlington, VA 22207; (800) 783-2240; www.medsports.com.

Hapad Arch Pads Hapad makes several pads that can relieve the discomfort of plantar fasciitis. The Longitudinal Metatarsal Arch Pads provide a corrective action that strengthens the longitudinal and metatarsal arches without restricting the natural flexibility of the foot. These pads may also help flat feet. The 3-Way Heel/Arch/Metatarsal Insoles is an all-in-one Longitudinal Metatarsal Arch Cushion and heel cushion which relieves plantar fasciitis and foot fatigue by supporting the arch, cushioning the heel and distributing pressure across the ball of the foot. The Comf-Orthotic 3/4-Length Insole is a contoured one-piece arch, metatarsal, and heel cushion that helps support flat feet. The coiled, spring-like wool fibers provide a firm and resilient support as they mold and shape to the foot. For more information contact Hapad Inc., PO Box 6, 5301 Enterprise Blvd., Bethel Park, PA 15102; (800) 544-2723; www.hapad.com.

Lynco Biomechanical Orthotic Systems Apex offers the Lynco Biomechanical Orthotic System, a "ready-made" triple-density orthotic system that comes in enough variations to accommodate 90% of foot disorders, including plantar fasciitis. See the chapter *Orthotics* on page 115 for information about Lynco orthotics.

N'ice Stretch Night Splint Suspension System Made for plantar fasciitis and Achilles tendinitis, this night splint uses bilateral suspension straps to provide continuous night time stretching of the plantar fasciitis and Achilles tendon. The straps allow for independent bi-plane dorsiflexion adjustment. A removable Sealed Ice pack provides cold therapy coupled with stretching of soft tissues. The unit is hinged to fold compactly. For more information contact Brown Medical Industries, 1300 Lundberg Drive West, Spirit Lake, IA 51360; (800) 843-4395; www.brownmed.com.

PF Night Splint AliMed makes four models of night splints to relieve the pain of plantar fasciitis. The PF Night Splint is a lightweight plastic splint designed to lessen morning pain caused by contractures and muscle tightening while sleeping. It is set at 5° dorsiflexion (the toes are 5° past 90°). The PF Night Splint II is a deluxe, terry cloth lined model which adjusts from 10° dorsiflexion to 10° plantar flexion (it comes preset at 5° dorsiflexion). The Early Fit Night Splint is fixed at 90° while the Early Fit Adjustable Night Splint can be set from 10° dorsiflexion to 40° plantar flexion. All splints fit both right or left feet and include a liner and straps to protect the leg and instep from pressure. An extra-wide model of the PF Night Splint is offered for those individuals with larger calves and ankles. For more information contact AliMed Inc., 297 High Street, Dedham, MA 02026-9135; (800) 225-2610; www.alimed.com.

Plantar reFLEX Night Splint   The Plantar reFLEX night splint is made for those wanting to wear a splint at night to help control their plantar fasciitis pain. The splint is adjustable and padded, with a breathable, replaceable, and washable Coolfoam liner. It comfortably positions the foot in a controlled amount of dorsiflexion enabling the application of Low Load Prolonged Stretch (LLPS) to the soft tissues of the plantar fascia and Achilles tendon. For more information contact Plantar reFLEX at (800) 922-8478, www.plantareflex.com.

Power*step* Insoles   The Power*step* insoles was design by a Dr. Les Appel to provide complete heel and arch support and stability. Its strong heel cradle prevents the foot from pronating (rolling inward) or the arch from flattening—eliminating strain on the plantar fascia. For more information contact Power*step*, PO Box 46744, Cincinnati, OH 46744; (888) 237-3668; www.powerstep.com.

ProStretch   This popular tool effectively stretches the plantar fascia, the Achilles tendon, and the calf muscles. The ProStretch builds lower extremity strength, balance, and flexibility benefits in three minutes of use prior to activity, thus reducing the risk of injury. The PT100 is unilateral while the PT200 is bilateral. Both models can also be used for hamstring and anterior tibialis stretching. For more information contact ProStretch at Prism Enterprises, 6952 Fairgrounds Parkway, San Antonio, TX 78238; (800) 535-3629; www.prostretch.com.

PSC - Pronation/Spring Control The PSC is a Pronation/Spring Control device. It is designed to treat plantar fasciitis, chronic heel pain, heel spur syndrome, and shin splints. This reusable strapping device is made from an open-celled, elastomeric, non-latex foam. It breathes to wick away perspiration, stays put with superior sticking power, and is fully adjustable. It wraps around the arch to provide superior support to the plantar fascia while also wrapping around the heel to reduce the force of heel strike and biomechanically move the foot's mid-line to a more neutral position. For more information contact fabrifoam Products, 900 Springdale Drive, Exton, PA 19341; (800) 577-1077; www.fabrifoam.com.

Strassburg Sock This unique sock is easy to use at night or extended periods of rest. A good alternative to the typical night splint, this system can be easily used and carried while backpacking. A standard over-the-calf tube sock uses two adjustable straps, one around the calf just below the knee, the other attached to the toe of the sock and passed through a "D" ring on the upper strap. Tension on the toe strap keeps the plantar fascia in a neutral to slightly stretched position, eliminating in the reduction or elimination of pain under the heel during initial weight bearing in the morning. For more information contact JT Enterprises LLC, PO Box 1253, N. Tonawanda, NY 14120; (800) 452-0631; www.thesock.com.

The Ultimate Heel & Arch Support Made by footcare specialist, Dr. G. Budak, the Ultimate is made from Visco Elastic Polymer that molds to the foot, forms a deep heel cup, and follows the contour of the arch, thereby making a custom fit. As a 3/4-length orthotic, it provides relief from plantar fasciitis, heel spur pain, Achilles tendonitis, and arch, knee, and back strain. It also absorbs up to 90% of shock which reduces stress to the heel, foot, leg, and back. For more information contact The Foot Store, 1909 N. Highway 17, Mount Pleasant, SC 29464; (800) 775-3668; www.footstore.com.

Viscoped S The Viscoped "S" insoles are made from a non-compressible, viscoelastic material with a bar of softer silicon in the metatarsal and heel areas. The insoles reduce shock throughout the entire length of the insole and distributes pressure evenly. Designed to relieve plantar fascia pain. For more information contact Bauerfeind USA, Inc., 2100 Barrett Park Drive, Suite 508, Kennesaw, GA 30144; (800) 423-3405; www.bauerfeind.com. Available through distributors or from Medco Sports Medicine (see page 273).

30

Achilles Tendinitis

The Achilles tendon is actually a cord that runs from the calf muscle downward to the back of the heel. The tendon makes it possible for you to rise up on your toes, run, and jump. Achilles tendinitis occurs when the sheath surrounding this cord becomes inflamed. Sudden and repeated stretching of the tendon can cause an inflammation that can produce pain behind the heel, ankle, and lower calf while walking and running. The pain may be felt during the early part of your run or hike, then subside, only to worsen after stopping. This pain is your first warning, followed by swelling of the Achilles tendon and pain to touch at the base of your heel.

A mild first-degree injury makes it difficult to rise up on your toes or walk on your heels. With proper treatment, you should be able to walk, with little pain, after about 48-hours. You should not resume normal athletic activity for several weeks. A second-degree injury is when there is partial tearing of the tendon from its attachment point. This injury will take from six to eight weeks to heal, with an additional two to four weeks of stretching exercises before normal athletic activity can be resumed. In a third-degree injury, an extreme case, the Achilles tendon ruptures. This requires immediate medical intervention, usually surgery, and a long healing and strengthening process.

A sudden increase in activity, increas-

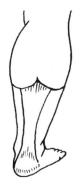

Achilles tendon

ing your mileage too fast, or running steep hills can lead to an inflamed Achilles tendon. To prevent Achilles tendon problems, increase your activity, mileage, and hill training gradually. Proper lower leg muscle stretching can also help prevent problems.

Rich Schick, a Physician's Assistant adds, "The Achilles tendon is not a simple structure, it is more correctly termed the Achilles complex. If it were as simple as we perceive it, there would be a straight pull from the calf muscle to the heel and the tendon would be very prominent instead of following the contour of the leg. In reality the tendon passes through a series of little tunnels of very tough tissue that hold it close to the leg.

In severe cases of Achilles tendonitis calcium deposits can form in and on the tendon preventing it from passing through these little tunnels and resulting in a permanent disability or the need for surgery. This is called calcific tendonitis. If you grasp the tendon between your thumb and forefinger, move your foot up and down, and feel a grating or bubble popping sensation this is a sign of serious tendonitis. The finding is called crepitus and represents severe inflammation. If not treated appropriately it can lead to calcific tendonitis. You must stop using the leg as much as possible, some authorities recommend casting, until this goes away. Ice and anti-inflammatory medication are also helpful."

Treatments

Treatment may include any or all of the following: icing as described below, stretching and flexibility exercises, wearing flexible shoes or boots with a well-padded heel counter, and avoiding the ups and downs of hills. Stop running—do not run through the pain. Ignoring the symptoms may cause the tendon to rupture, which usually requires surgery. Call your orthopedist or podiatrist if the pain persists. The doctor may put your foot in either a flexible or immobilizing cast to reduce movement and weight bearing. Once the cast is removed, you will need to do stretching exercises to strengthen the tendon before resuming normal athletic activity.

The treatment for a mildly injured Achilles tendinitis is the same RICE treatment used for ankle sprains and strains. R = rest,

I = ice, C = compression, and E = elevation. The first 24 hours are the most critical for beginning treatment. Early treatment decreases swelling and lessens the risk of additional injury. Initial rest of the foot is also important. A lightly wrapped Ace wrap will provide compression to help keep swelling down while providing support. Apply the Ace wrap from the forefoot upwards towards the calf. Do not wear the Ace wrap to bed at night. Apply ice for 20 minutes at a time three to four times daily. Ice can be very helpful in the healing process. Refer to the chapter on *Cold & Heat Therapy* on page 257 for more information on making the most of icing techniques. The injured area should be elevated above the level of the heart as much as possible during the first 48 hours. This keeps blood away from the injured area and reduces pain and swelling. The use of anti-inflammatory medications is usually warranted.

Since ligaments and tendons do not have their own direct blood supply, their healing is slow. Karl King found that the nutritional supplements of one gram Glycine, one gram Lysine, one-half gram buffered Vitamin C, and one Aleve tablet is helpful in the healing process. While he recommends these supplements for an ankle sprain, they might also help an inflamed Achilles tendon. Take this combination at breakfast and at bedtime. The supplements provide the major building blocks for connective tissue while the Aleve is an anti-inflammatory.

A small heel pad will alleviate the stresses on the tendon. For some individuals, wearing low-heeled shoes as often as possible will help keep the Achilles tendon stretched. An Achilles notch in shoes or mid- and low-top boots will accommodate the Achilles tendon in plantar flexion. The Achilles Tendon Strap made by Cho-Pat can provide relief from the discomfort of Achilles tendinitis.

A lightweight plastic night splint worn to bed can help to stretch the foot, limit contraction of soft tissues at night, and avoid morning stiffness. Night splints help avoid footdrop and accompanying muscle tightening. Night splints are proven as a treatment method of preventing the plantar fascia and Achilles tendon from contracting during the night. Many athletes swear by them. Check with your podiatrist, orthopedist, or medical supply store. Several night splint models are available. The Strassburg Sock is an alternative style night splint which can be worn at night or while resting to lightly stretch the plantar fascia.

If the pain persists, consult a medical specialist. They will need to rule out partial tears of the tendon, an inflammation of the tendon's sheath, or degenerative changes.

Stretching Exercises

Stretching helps athletes improve flexibility and counter muscular imbalances that puts them at a greater risk of injury. Proper stretching of the Achilles tendon can help prevent an Achilles injury.

- One method of stretching is to stand far enough from a wall or heavy piece of furniture so that when you lean forward towards the wall or furniture you can feel the tendons stretch in the back of your leg while keeping your feet flat on the floor. Lean forward and stretch only to the point of feeling the stretch, not to the point of feeling pain. Alternate a 20 seconds stretch with a 20 rest standing straight, repeated ten to twenty times. Continue this daily stretching until the Achilles stops hurting.

- Dr. Les Appel, who designed the Power*step* Insole recommends facing a wall with one foot flat on the floor and the other foot's heel on the floor and toes up on the wall 3-4 inches. Gently move your knee slowly towards the wall until you feel slight stretching on the bottom of your foot and the back of your leg. Hold this position for 30 seconds, repeating five times per foot.

- A Swedish study showed excellent results with a simple stretch. Stand on a step or ledge on the balls of your feet. Push yourself up with your good leg and slowly transfer your weight to the affected leg. Slowly lower yourself all the way down until the injured leg's heel is below the stair level and you feel the pull on the soleus calf muscle. Alternated this stretch with the injured leg's knee straight and then slightly bent. Repeat three sets of 15 times each, twice a day. Additional strength can be gained by adding weight over time. Use dumbbells, a light barbell, or a weighted backpack.

The ProStretch is a popular tool to effectively stretch the plantar fascia as well as the Achilles tendon and the gastrocnemius and soleus musculature of the back of the lower leg. Studies have shown that utilization of the ProStretch can more effectively increase ankle dorsiflexion (toe-up motion of the ankle) than by the conventional and commonly used wall stretch technique mentioned above.[28] Its use is recommended as both a preventive measure as well as a treatment technique.

Products

Achilles Strap   A new Achilles strap is in the developmental stage. Check the fabrifoam web site for product release information or contact fabrifoam Products, 900 Springdale Drive, Exton, PA 19341; (800) 577-1077; www.fabrifoam.com.

Cho-Pat Achilles Tendon Strap   Cho-Pat makes this Achilles tendon strap which fits under the arch and around the ankle to relieve pressure on the Achilles tendon. Trials at the Mayo's Sports/Medicine Clinic have shown the strap effective as an addition to traditional treatment procedures for Achilles tendinitis, particularly during the push-off phase of gait. The strap is available in four sizes based on ankle circumference at its widest point. For more information contact Cho-Pat, Inc. PO Box 293, Hainesport, NJ 08036; (800) 221-1601; www.cho-pat.com.

Hapad Heel Pads   Hapad makes the 3/4-Length Heel Wedges that provides necessary heel lift to help reduce the pain associated with Achilles tendinitis. It is available in three thicknesses. The coiled, spring-like wool fibers provide firm and resilient support as they mold and shape to the foot. For more information contact Hapad Inc., PO Box 6, 5301 Enterprise Blvd., Bethel Park, PA 15102; (800) 544-2723; www.hapad.com.

N'ice Stretch Night Splint Suspension System
Made for plantar fasciitis and Achilles tendinitis, this night splint uses bilateral suspension straps to provide continuous night time stretching of the plantar fasciitis and Achilles tendon. The straps allow for independent bi-plane dorsiflexion adjustment. A removable Sealed Ice pack provides cold therapy coupled with stretch-

ing of soft tissues. The unit is hinged to fold compactly. For more information contact Brown Medical Industries, 1300 Lundberg Drive West, Spirit Lake, IA 51360; (800) 843-4395; www.brownmed.com.

Plantar reFLEX Night Splint   The   Plantar reFLEX night splint is made for those wanting to wear a splint at night to help control their plantar fasciitis pain. The splint is adjustable and padded, with a breathable, replaceable, and washable Coolfoam liner. It comfortably positions the foot in a controlled amount of dorsiflexion enabling the application of Low Load Prolonged Stretch (LLPS) to the soft tissues of the plantar fascia and Achilles tendon. For more information contact Plantar reFLEX at (800) 922-8478, www.plantareflex.com.

ProStretch   This popular tool effectively stretches the Achilles tendon, the plantar fiscia, and the calf muscles. The ProStretch builds lower extremity strength, balance, and flexibility benefits in three minutes of use prior to activity, thus reducing the risk of injury. The PT100 is unilateral while the PT200 is bilateral. Both models can also be used for hamstring and anterior tibialis stretching. For more information contact ProStretch at Prism Enterprises, 6952 Fairgrounds Parkway, San Antonio, TX 78238; (800) 535-3629; www.prostretch.com.

Strassburg Sock   This unique sock is easy to use at night or extended periods of rest. A good alternative to the typical night splint, this system can be easily used and carried while backpacking. A standard over-the-calf tube sock uses two adjustable straps, one around the calf just below the knee, the other attached to the toe of the sock and passed through a "D" ring on the upper strap. Tension on the toe strap keeps the plantar fascia in a neutral to slightly stretched position, eliminating in the reduction or elimination of pain under the heel during initial weight bearing in the morning. For more information contact JT Enterprises LLC, PO Box 1253, N. Tonawanda, NY 14120; (800) 452-0631; www.thesock.com.

31

Stubbed Toes & Toenail Problems

Stubbed Toes

Occasionally we stub our toes resulting in a hematoma, a bruise, or even a fracture. Stubbed toes are more common in running shoes than in hiking boots. Stubbing a toe on a rock or tree root can be very painful. Check the toe for discoloration that can indicate a deep bruise or a fracture. There may be a laceration into the nailbed or into the toe itself.

Treatments

Treatment includes "buddy taping," icing the toe (a cold stream will also work), elevation, and a firm soled shoe or boot. Buddy taping is done by lightly taping the injured toe to the toe next to it, with a piece of cotton between (never tape skin-to-skin). Buddy taping provides support and a limited degree of immobilization to the toe. A firm soled shoe will keep the toe from bending, providing additional immobilization. For elevation to be effective, the injured toe should be above the level of the heart.

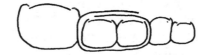

With cotton between toes, lightly tape the injured toe to a good toe

If it heals in a few days, it is likely not fractured. On the other hand, if the injury does not respond to treatment, medical treatment and an x-ray may be necessary. A doctor may have you wear an orthopedic shoe, a wooden soled shoe that does not allow the foot to bend. If the toe is fractured, expect a healing time of four to six weeks. See page 257 on *Cold & Heat Therapy* for more information on making the most of icing techniques. If a fracture is suspected, see the section on *Fractures* on page 194.

Toenail Problems

All athletes need to maintain good toenail care. Toenails should be trimmed regularly, straight across the nail—never rounded at the corners. After trimming toenails, use a nail file to smooth the top of the nail down toward the front of the toe and remove any rough edges. If you draw your finger from the skin in front of the toe up across the nail and can feel a rough edge, the nail can be filed smoother or trimmed a bit shorted. Remember though, the shorter your nails are trimmed the more likelihood you will have an ingrown toenail. Leave an extra bit of nail on the outside corner of the big toe to avoid an ingrown toenail. Shoes that are too tight in the forefoot or too short can cause the nail to press into the sides of the toe.

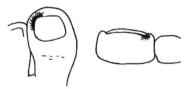

Ingrown toenail, most common on the big toe

Ingrown toenails, most common to the big toe, may cause infection and require medical attention. One or both sides of your toenail may grow into the flesh of the toe. The result is a reddened, irritated, and swollen toe that is sensitive to any degree of pressure. These are usually very painful and require immediate attention.

The technical name for the runner's black toenail, "subungal hematoma," is simply a blood-filled swelling under the nail. This common occurrence is caused by the trauma of the toe or toes repetitively bumping against the front of the shoe. Individuals with Morton's Foot are most susceptible to having black toenails. The nail becomes discolored and usually has associated pain.

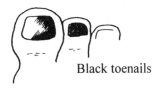

Black toenails

Treatments

Soak your foot in warm water or Epsom Salts two to three times a day to reduce the infection. Do not poke at the ingrown nail. If you cannot trim the nail yourself, check with your orthopedist or podiatrist. An ignored ingrown toenail can become seriously infected. Apply a layer of antibiotic cream to help reduce inflammation and cover with a Band-Aid.

Rich Schick, PA, recommends the following method to care for an ingrown nail. "File the entire top surface of the nail from near the cuticle to the tip until you get it as thin as possible. A regular nail file will work but a medium grade metal file is much quicker. This weakens the nail. Then soak the foot in hot water for about thirty minutes to soften the nail, further weakening the nail. Then use a cuticle trimmer (available in most drugstore beauty departments) to free the ingrown portion. Do not attempt to work from the tip towards the base. Come from the side, and a little towards the base of the toe and use the "wings" of the instrument to lift and free the ingrown segment. Continuing forward the trimmer will often cut the piece off. If not snip it with a nail clipper. I prefer a small pair of wire cutters for the task."

To relieve pressure from a black toenail, use one of the following methods depending on the look of the toenail. The treatment may have to be repeated several times. Although the two methods below might sound painful, they are usually not painful.

- If the discoloration does not extend to the end of the toenail, swab the nail with an alcohol wipe, and use a small drill bit or hypodermic needle to gently drill a hole in the nail with light pressure and rolling the needle/bit back and forth between your thumb and fingers. The blood will ooze through the hole. Keep slight pressure on the nail bed to help expel the built-up blood. Stopping too soon will cause the blood to clot in the hole and the problem will reoccur.
- An alternative method is to use a match to heat a pin, needle, or in a pinch, a paper clip, and gently penetrate the nail with the heated point. The heat in this method can cauterize the blood stop the flow of blood out from under the nail.
- If the discoloration extends to the end of the toenail, use a sterile pin or needle to penetrate the skin under the nail and release the pressure. Holding slight pressure on the nail bed will help expel the blood.

Care must be taken to prevent a secondary bacterial infection through the hole in the nail or at the end of the nail by using an antibiotic ointment and covering the site with a Band-Aid. Loss of the nail usually follows in the months ahead. The new nail will begin growing, pushing up the old nail and may come in looking odd. Do not be concerned about the process unless an infection develops. Dr. David Hannaford, a podiatrist, tells of patients who come to see him thinking they "... have cancer because their nails are growing in funny looking."

Many runners are simply prone to black toenails. Some runners choose to have them surgically removed. The best means of preventing black toenails is to wear shoes with a generous toe box and the proper length for your feet. Paul Vorwerk used to think shoes should fit tight "... like a surgeon's glove," but after losing nails on his big toes, he now runs in shoes with good toe space. Some runners cut slits in their shoe's toe box or cut out a portion of the toe box to gain relief. "When I have any toenails at all, I use moleskin." reports Jim Winne who has perpetually black toenails. His strategy is to cut a piece of moleskin slightly larger than the nail area, put it on the nail, and round the edges. Use an alcohol wipe on the nail before applying and be sure the moleskin does not rub on adjoining toes. Duct tape and Elastikon tape would also work.

You may find relief by wearing a metatarsal pad, a small circular pad that pushes up the ball of the foot and drops the toes down, which takes pressure off the toenails. Contact Hapad Inc. for information on these pads.

If you stub your toe and the nail is bent backwards, the key is to prevent the toenail from catching on your sock and tearing off. Wrap either a Band-Aid or tape around the toe to hold the toenail in place. The use of an antibiotic ointment under the nail will help prevent infection.

Fungus under and around the nails should be treated promptly with antifungal medications. See the chapter *Athlete's Foot* on page 253 for information on treating fungal infections.

Products

Assorted Products   Check your local drug store and pharmacy for a current selection of related products. A sampling includes: Dr. Scholl's Ingrown Toenail Relief Strips.

FootSmart   FootSmart carries a complete line of skin care products made for the feet. Several products are made for nail care. For information on the following products contact FootSmart Products, PO Box 922908, Norcross, GA 30010; (800) 870-7149; www.footsmart.com.

- The Barrel Nipper is a long-handled nail clippers made for thick, tough, curved nails.
- Toenail Softening Cream is made with a toenail softening agent.
- Ingrown Toenail File

32

Morton's Foot & Hammer Toes

Morton's Foot

Morton's foot is a common problem where second toe (next to the big toe) is longer than the big toe. The first metatarsal (of the big toe) is shorter than normal and this makes the second toe appear longer than it actually is. The repeated pressure of the longer second toe against the front of the shoe or boot may traumatize the nail. If a hematoma develops under the nail, the nail will change color and may fall off. This is usually a hereditary condition. Morton's Foot is often associated with Metatarsalgia.

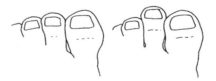

Morton's foot is when the first
toe is longer than the big toe

Treatments

To get a good fit, look for shoes or boots with a wide toe box. It may be necessary to use a shoe or boot one or more sizes larger than normal in order to have space for the longer first toe. The use of a non-slippery insole will keep the foot from sliding forward. Look for an insole with a good heel cup, an arch that fits your foot, and a surface material that grips the foot and sock. Some runners will cut a slit over or on either side of the toe to relieve pressure. Another option is to cut out a small piece of the toe box over the toe. Orthotics may also provide relief. Surgery is usually a last resort.

Hammer Toes

Hammer toes are toes that are contracted at the toe's middle joint, making the toe bend upward at its center and forcing the tip of the toe downward. The ligaments and tendons have tightened and are forcing the curl effect. This can lead to severe pressure and pain. Hammer toes can occur in any toe, except the big toe. There are two types of hammer toes—rigid and flexible. A rigid toe has no ability to move whereas in the flexible toe the joint can be moved. Hammer toes result when a muscle imbalance causes the ligaments and tendons to tighten. Individuals with flat feet are more prone to hammer toes, calluses and bunions.

Treatments

Changing footwear to a style that offers a high and broad toe box. This usually allows the other toes additional room so there is less friction against the individual toes. Corrective surgery is often the only option.

Products

Assorted Products   Check your local drug store and pharmacy for a current selection of related products. A sampling includes: Dr. Scholl's Hammer Toe Pads.

FootSmart   FootSmart carries the Silicone Toe Crest that fits over one toe and "nestles" under the hammer toe for support while reliving pressure and friction. The Toe Straightener properly aligns hammer toes (also in a Double Toe model). Gel Toe Separators and/or the Gel Toe Spreader may also provide relief. For information on these products contact FootSmart Products, PO Box 922908, Norcross, GA 30010; (800) 870-7149; www.footsmart.com.

33

Metatarsalgia, Morton's Neuroma, & Sesamoiditis

Metatarsalgia

Metatarsalgia is pain underneath the metatarsal heads of the foot. It typically occurs when one of the metatarsal heads collapses and points downward. Typically the second metatarsal head is affected, but it can also be at the third or fourth metatarsal heads. It may feel like there is a small stone in your shoe; or pain, burning sensation or swelling at the ball of the foot. By pressing up slightly on each metatarsal head you can usually identify the painful area. Typically the metatarsal head that is lower then the others is causing the pain and pressure. There often will be a callus at the pressure point. As we age, the fat pads on the bottoms of our feet tend to thin out and our feet become more susceptible to this problem. Metatarsalgia is often associated with Morton's Foot.

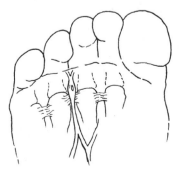

A nerve inflammation indicating Morton's neuroma

Shoes that are to narrow in the forefoot and/or lacing too tight over the forefoot area can cause all of these problems. Grasp your foot at the base of the toes and squeeze gently. See how it forces the metatarsals downward and results in increased impact to the area with each step.

Treatments

A cushioned metatarsal pad can provide relief from metatarsalgia. If the pad does not help, try cutting a small hole in the insole under the painful metatarsal head. Wearing shoes with a wide forefoot and high and wide toe box is also recommended. An orthotic may be necessary. For proper prevention, start with shoes that fit correctly and incorporate See the sections *Getting a Proper Fit* on page 38 and the *Lacing Options* chapter on page 139.

Products

FootSmart   FootSmart carries a Silicone Ball-of-Foot Cushion that redistributes pressure on the metatarsal heads. For information contact FootSmart Products, PO Box 922908, Norcross, GA 30010; (800) 870-7149; www.footsmart.com.

Hapad Pads   Hapad makes several pads to use for these problems. Metatarsal Pads relieve the pain of metatarsalgia and Morton's neuroma. Metatarsal Bars relieve pressure on the ball of the foot that causes painful calluses and forefoot irritations. Metatarsal Cookies provide simple metatarsal arch cushioning. The coiled, spring-like wool fibers provide firm and resilient support as they mold and shape to the foot. For more information contact Hapad Inc., PO Box 6, 5301 Enterprise Blvd., Bethel Park, PA 15102; (800) 544-2723; www.hapad.com.

Spenco Cushions   Spenco makes a Metatarsal Arch Cushion for the ball of the foot and an Arch Cushion for better arch support. For more information contact Spenco Medical Corporation, PO Box 2501, Waco, TX 76702-2501; (800) 877-3626; www.spenco.com.

Viscoped   The regular Viscoped insoles are made from a non-compressible, viscoelastic material with areas of softer density in the raised metatarsal head pad and heel areas. The Viscoped "S" insole is made with bar of softer silicon in the metatarsal and heel areas. The insoles reduce shock throughout the entire length of the insole and distribute pressure evenly. Made to relieve pain associated with metatarsalgia and Morton's neuroma. For more information contact Bauerfeind USA, Inc., 2100 Barrett Park Drive, Suite 508, Kennesaw, GA 30144; (800) 423-3405; www.bauerfeind.com. Available through distributors or from Medco Sports Medicine (see page 273).

Morton's Neuroma

Morton's Neuroma is pain associated with a nerve inflammation usually affecting the third and fourth toes. The nerves running between the metatarsal heads and the toes have become inflamed and irritated as they are squeezed at the base of the toes. There is typically tingling, burning, or a pins-and-needles sensation that radiates to the end of the toes. If untreated, scar tissue forms around the nerve and it becomes more painful.

This can be caused by a shoe's tight toe box, compressing the forefoot, or by the nerves being pressured by the metatarsal heads and the bases of the toes. Sports that place a significant amount of pressure on the forefoot area can make the nerves become inflammed.

Treatments

Treatments include applying ice to the pain area, an injection of anti-inflammatory medication, wider shoes, a more cushioned insole, and metatarsal pads that take pressure off the metatarsal heads. Removing the shoe and massaging the foot usually relieves the pain.

If you over-pronate, the metatarsal bones have more movement which can irritate the nerves running between the metatarsal heads. In this case, wearing firm motion-control shoes may help. Relief may also be gained by inserting a piece of lamb's wool between the toes. The use of an orthotic may be indicated. Bursitis, bunions, or arthritis may also cause metatarsal pain. Your podiatrist or orthopedist can help identify the cause of the pain and make recommendations on how to treat the problems. Serious neuromas may require surgery to release or remove the affected nerve. Ice according to recommendation in *Cold & Heat Therapy* on page 257.

To relieve pressure on the metatarsal heads and forefoot, try different lacing techniques. Use one pair of laces per shoe. Lace one through the bottom half of the eyelets tied loosely. Lace the other through the top half of the eyelets tied more tightly than the bottom lace. Another method, recommended by Steve Pero, is to lace the first few loops loosely, tie a knot, and then lace the rest of the way up the shoe. With these methods the metatarsal heads are not squeezed by the pressure of normal lacing. The chapter *Lacing Options* on page 139 describes more lacing techniques.

Strengthening Exercises

Toe exercises help to strengthen and tighten the metatarsal arch and stretch the tendons on top of the toes. Practice picking up marbles with your toes. Put a towel on the floor and use your toes to scrunch up the towel and pick it up.

Products

FootSmart   FootSmart carries a Silicone Ball-of-Foot Cushion that redistributes pressure on the metatarsal heads. For information contact FootSmart Products, PO Box 922908, Norcross, GA 30010; (800) 870-7149; www.footsmart.com.

Hapad Pads   Hapad makes several pads to use for these problems. Metatarsal Pads relieve the pain of metatarsalgia and Morton's neuroma. Metatarsal Bars relieve pressure on the ball of the foot that causes painful calluses and forefoot irritations. Metatarsal Cookies provide simple metatarsal arch cushioning. The coiled, spring-like wool fibers provide firm and resilient support as they mold and shape to the foot. For more information contact Hapad Inc., PO Box 6, 5301 Enterprise Blvd., Bethel Park, PA 15102; (800) 544-2723; www.hapad.com.

Spenco Cushions   Spenco makes a Metatarsal Arch Cushion for the ball of the foot and an Arch Cushion for better arch support. For more information contact Spenco Medical Corporation, PO Box 2501, Waco, TX 76702-2501; (800) 877-3626; www.spenco.com.

Viscoped   The regular Viscoped insoles are made from a non-compressible, viscoelastic material with areas of softer density in the raised metatarsal head pad and heel areas. The Viscoped "S" insole is made with bar of softer silicon in the metatarsal and heel areas. The insoles reduce shock throughout the entire length of the insole and distribute pressure evenly. Made to relieve pain associated with metatarsalgia and Morton's neuroma. For more information contact Bauerfeind USA, Inc., 2100 Barrett Park Drive, Suite 508, Kennesaw, GA 30144; (800) 423-3405; www.bauerfeind.com. Available through distributors or from Medco Sports Medicine (see page 273).

Sesamoiditis

Sesamoiditis is an inflammation of the two little bones beneath the ball of the foot, under the joint that moves the big toe. These two sesamoid bones can become bruised and inflamed, resulting in sharp pain. The bones can also fracture.

Rich Schick, a Physician's Assistant, points out that the sesamoid under the first metatarsal is often composed of several small bones. He says, "If the bones on an x-ray were smooth appearing with no rough or jagged edges, this is likely the situation. Even if it is a fracture, these bones only act as shock absorbers in the first place. One can continue to run with nothing to fear but pain. I high centered on a sharp rock a some years back and fractured mine. On x-ray there were two pieces like half moons with the round side smooth and the straight sides jagged as one would expect if you broke a round object in half. The literature said that these fractures could lead to chronic pain and the fragments could need to be surgically removed. As this 'worse case' didn't seem all that frightening I opted to train and race as normal. The thing bothered me for about a year but for the last several years gives me no pain at all."

These two little bones can became a major problem. Lyal Holmberg experienced a sesamoid problem after when the ball of his left foot became painful after a short five-mile run. An X-ray showed the sesamoid bone was broken into three pieces. Lyal reports that, "As I continued running, the foot was killing me and caused a tilt towards the right, putting a strain on my left hip." A walking-type boot and an anti-inflammatory was prescribed for two weeks, then the use of a small "dancer's" pad behind the ball of my foot while trying to walk and run. Lyal says, "If I can walk and run without pain, then the problem is solved. If not, I may need surgery to correct the problem."

Treatments

The use of soft pads or insoles can help. You can also cut a small hole in your insole under the sesamoid bones. Loosely lacing the forefoot of your shoes, as described above, can help relieve pressure on the sesamoid area. Using icing techniques from the chapter *Cold & Heat Therapy* on page 257 can help reduce pain and inflammation.

Products

Hapad Pads   Hapad makes Dancer Pads that fit under the ball of the foot with a cutout encompassing the big toe joint to relieve calluses and the painful irritations of sesamoiditis. The coiled, spring-like wool fibers provide firm and resilient support as they mold and shape to the foot. For more information contact Hapad Inc., PO Box 6, 5301 Enterprise Blvd., Bethel Park, PA 15102; (800) 544-2723; www.hapad.com.

Spenco Cushions   Spenco makes a Metatarsal Arch

Cushion for the ball of the foot and an Arch Cushion for better arch support. For more information contact Spenco Medical Corporation, PO Box 2501, Waco, TX 76702-2501; (800) 877-3626; www.spenco.com.

Viscoped   The regular Viscoped insoles are made from a non-compressible, viscoelastic material with areas of softer density in the raised metatarsal head pad and heel areas. The Viscoped "S" insole is made with bar of softer silicon in the metatarsal and heel areas. The insoles reduce shock throughout the entire length of the insole and distribute pressure evenly. Made to relieve pain associated with metatarsalgia and Morton's neuroma. For more information contact Bauerfeind USA, Inc., 2100 Barrett Park Drive, Suite 508, Kennesaw, GA 30144; (800) 423-3405; www.bauerfeind.com. Available through distributors or from Medco Sports Medicine (see page 273).

34

Corns, Calluses, Bunions, & Bursitis

Corns

A corn is a hard, thickened area of skin, generally on the top of, the tip of, or between the toes, usually caused by friction and pressure. A corn is usually, like a kernel of corn, round and yellowish in color. Corns on the outer surface of the toes are usually hard while those between the toes are usually soft. The larger the corn and the more it rubs against your shoe, the more painful it becomes.

The causes of corns can be tight fitting socks and footwear, deformed toes, or the foot sliding around the shoe. Soft corns are caused by bony prominences and are found between the toes—soft from the perspiration in the forefoot area.

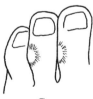

Corns

Treatments

To relieve the discomfort of corns, start with properly fitting shoes with extra room in the toe box. You can also try corn pads, small pieces of one of the tapes previously mentioned, or Spenco 2nd Skin. Lamb's wool can be wrapped around the toe for cushioning. There are many types of corn pads and toe sleeves. Check the footcare section of your local drug store for a current selection of corn relief products.

To control corns, the pressure and friction must be eliminated, usually from improper fitting shoes. To relieve pressure on the painful area, try different lacing techniques. Use one pair of laces per shoe. Lace one through the bottom half of the eyelets tied loosely. Lace the other through the top half of the eyelets tied more tightly than the bottom lace. A second method is to lace the first few loops loosely, tie a knot, and then lace the rest of the way up the shoe. Both methods allow a looser fit in the forefoot.

Products

Assorted Products　　Check your local drug store and pharmacy for a current selection of related products. A sampling includes: Band-Aid Corn Relief, Dr. Scholl's Corn Cushions, Dr. Scholl's Moisturizing Corn Remover Kit, and Dr. Scholl's Waterproof Corn Cushions, FreeZone Corn and Callus Remover, and FreeZone One-Step Corn Remover Pads.

Hapad Pads　　Hapad makes several pads to use for these problems. Metatarsal Cookies provide simple metatarsal arch cushioning which can relieve the pressure that causes corns and calluses. The coiled, spring-like wool fibers provide firm and resilient support as they mold and shape to the foot. For more information contact Hapad Inc., PO Box 6, 5301 Enterprise Blvd., Bethel Park, PA 15102; (800) 544-2723; www.hapad.com.

FootSmart　　FootSmart carries the Happy Feet Corn Salve with a Salicylic acid-based cream to remove corns. For information contact FootSmart Products, PO Box 922908, Norcross, GA 30010; (800) 870-7149; www.footsmart.com.

Calluses

A callus is an abnormal amount of dead, thickened skin caused by recurring pressure and friction, called *hyperkeratoses*, usually on the sole of the foot, most often on the heels, the balls of the feet or the bottom of the toes. Calluses can form over any bony prominence. Calluses are never normal, but are a sign of poor biomechanics or ill-fitting footgear. If it is a footgear problem this needs to be identified and remedied. Unfortunately most biomechanical problems are things we need to learn to live with. Calluses become a problem when they become thick enough

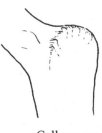

Calluses on the heel

to interfere with the normal elasticity of the skin or to act like a foreign body on the foot.

Unless the callus is troublesome, most people tend to forget about them. Your body has made the callus as protection from pressure at points with little natural fat or padding. To keep painful calluses from returning, you must correct the biomechanical problem that prompted their growth in the first place. Metatarsal bones that are too long or badly aligned, arches that are too high or too low, or a lessening of the fat pad on the heel can cause calluses. Some calluses may have a deep-seated core, called *nucleation*, that can be painful to pressure. These are called intractable plantar keratosis. These should be treated by a podiatrist.

Calluses are caused by a number of factors. Mal-aligned metatarsal bones in the forefoot, an abnormal gait, flat or high arched feet, excessively long metatarsal bones, and a loss of the fat pads on the underside of the foot. Individuals with flat feet are more prone to calluses, bunions, and hammer toes.

Calluses will continue to grow as they toughen. This can interfere with the fit of your shoes—which in turn can cause a blister—one way or another.

Treatments

Grasp some normal skin on your foot and roll it between your thumb and forefinger noticing how supple it is. Now attempt to roll the callused area in the same manner. If it is too stiff or causes discomfort the callus is too thick and is likely to cause pain or blisters. You need to thin it down. Simply keep working at it until all areas are as supple as normal skin.

Warm water and Epsom salt soaks and creams or lotions will help soften corns and calluses. Take a hot water foot soak and gently rub off any softened callused skin with a towel. After the callused skin is dry, apply your choice of cream, lotion, medication, or pads. Several foot files are available for use on calluses or use an emery board. Geraldine Wales has a tendency to get tough calluses on her feet that turn into hot spots and eventually blisters. In the evening she uses the file on the calluses and then applies moisturizing cream to keep her feet soft. Never file too deeply to cut into a corn or callus and do not cut into them with sharp objects. A pumice stone will work the same as the file.

A cushioned insole with a good arch support can help equalize the weight load of the foot while pads around or near the callus can relieve pressure. An orthotic may be necessary, either over-the-counter or custom made. To relieve heel discomfort, try a heel cup or heel pad that will distribute body weight evenly across the heel. The regular use of skin moisturizers will help keep the skin soft. To relieve pressure on the painful area, try different lacing techniques described in the *Corns* section of this chapter.

While there are over-the-counter plantar wart removal compounds available that can also be used on corns and calluses, care must be taken in their use. These products contain salicylic acid. Follow the product's directions to avoid damaging good tissue. Do not use these products if you are a diabetic. Check your local drug store or pharmacy for a complete line of products.

Products

Assorted Products   Check your local drug store and pharmacy for a current selection of related products. A sampling includes: Band-Aid Callus Relief, Dr. Scholl's Pedicure File, Dr. Scholl's Dual-Action Swedish File, Dr. School's Callus Reducer, Dr. Scholl's Callus Cushions, Dr. Scholl's Cushlin Gel Pads, and FreeZone Corn and Callus Remover.

Avon's Double Action Foot File   This foot file is 7″ long and has a coarse side and a fine side to remove dry skin buildup and calluses. It can be used on either wet or dry skin. After filing, apply a moisturizing cream. For more information contact Avon Products, 9 West 57th Street, NY, NY 10019; (800) FOR-AVON

Hapad Pads   Hapad makes several pads to use for these problems. Metatarsal Pads and Metatarsal Bars reduce pressure on the ball of the foot that causes painful calluses. Metatarsal Cookies provide simple metatarsal arch cushioning which can relieve the pressure that causes corns and calluses. Dancer Pads have a cut out encompassing the big toe joint to relieve calluses and painful irritations. Heel Cushions and Horseshoe Heel Cushions provide comfort from heel calluses. The coiled, spring-like wool fibers provide firm and resilient support as they mold and shape to the foot. For more information contact Hapad Inc., PO Box 6, 5301 Enterprise Blvd., Bethel Park, PA 15102; (800) 544-2723; www.hapad.com.

FootSmart   FootSmart carries a complete line of skin care products made for the feet. These products will help your feet feel softer and smoother while eliminating calluses. For information on the following products contact FootSmart Products, PO Box 922908, Norcross, GA 30010; (800) 870-7149; www.footsmart.com.

- Total Foot Recovery Cream/Lotion with Alpha Hydroxy Acid and deep-penetrating Urethin to soften dry and callused feet.
- Callus Treatment Cream with Urethin to break down painful, hardened skin.
- Dr. D's Foot and Heel Cream with Tea Tree Oil, 10% Aloe Vera, and Vitamin E.
- Heel Treatment Cream with Urethin and Aloe Vera.
- Lansinoh Cream with 100% lanolin for superior moisturizing properties.
- A Callus File to reduce thick calluses.

Bunions

Bunions are one of the most common deformities of the forefoot. A bunion is a bump caused by enlarged bone and tissue at the outer base of the big toe where the joint angles inward toward the other toes. A displacement of the first metatarsal bone towards the mid-line (center) of the body, and a simultaneous displacement of the big toe away from the mid-line (and towards the smaller toes) causes this bump to appear. A similar bump at the outer base of the fifth (small) toe is called a bunionette. Over time, the big toe can come to rest under, or occasionally over, the second toe. The bony bump is a form of arthritis.

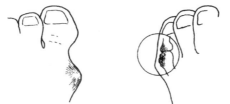

Bunion at the base of the big toe and bunionette on the little toe

The deformity gives you a wide-foot and causes a weakening and sagging of the arch. The motion of the joint and shoe pressure can cause pain. There may be corns on the adjacent sides of the first and second toes. A calluses may develop over the bunion, and bursitis can form between the skin and the bunion bone.

Bunions are caused by an various factors. An abnormal pronated foot that rolls inward, is one of the most common causes. Other causes include a family history of bunions, wearing shoes that are too narrow toed, and limb length discrepancy. Individuals with flat feet are more prone to bunions, calluses, and hammer toes.

Treatments

Be sure your shoes are wide and deep enough in the forefoot and toe box . If you over-pronate, try an arch support or orthotic to reduce the over-pronation. Bunion discomfort may be relieved with wider shoes, pads between the big and first toes, arch supports, and warm soaks. Check the footcare section of your local drug store for a current selection of bunion relief products. If there is an inflammation of the bunion, take an anti-inflammatory medication, elevate the foot, and apply ice three times a day, fifteen minutes at a time. For information on *Cold & Heat Therapy* techniques, see page 257. Surgery may be necessary in extreme cases.

A full service shoe shop or a pedorthist should be able to modify a boot to soften a pressure point or stretch a portion of the leather. This may relieve pressure on corns, calluses, and bunions. To relieve pressure on the painful area, try different lacing techniques described in the *Corns* section of this chapter.

Products

Assorted Products   Check your local drug store and pharmacy for a current selection of related products. A sampling includes: Dr. Scholl's Bunion Cushion Pads.

Hapad Pads   Hapad makes several pads to use for these problems. Metatarsal Pads and Metatarsal Bars reduce pressure on the ball of the foot that causes painful calluses. Metatarsal Cookies provide simple metatarsal arch cushioning which can relieve the pressure that causes corns and calluses. Dancer Pads have a cut out encompassing the big toe joint to relieve calluses and painful irritations. Heel Cushions and Horseshoe Heel Cushions provide comfort from heel calluses. The coiled, spring-like wool fibers provide firm and resilient support as they mold and shape to the foot. For more information contact Hapad Inc., PO Box 6, 5301 Enterprise Blvd., Bethel Park, PA 15102; (800) 544-2723; www.hapad.com.

FootSmart   FootSmart carries a complete line of skin care products made for the feet. Several of these products will help with bunion problems. For information contact FootSmart Products, PO Box 922908, Norcross, GA 30010; (800) 870-7149; www.footsmart.com.

- The Gel Toe Spreader and Gel Toe Separators are made of a soft patented gel with time-release mineral oil to relieve friction and irritation.
- The Bunion Comforter puts a cushioned ring of protection between your bunion and your shoe.

Bursitis

Bursae are small fluid-filled sacs found between areas of high friction such as bone against soft tissue or bone against a hard surface. The bursa acts as a shock absorber, allowing movement between neighboring structures. The body has more than 150 bursa sacs. Bursitis is the formation of an inflamed fluid-filled sac from trauma or overuse. On the feet, bursitis may develop beneath a callus or a bunion, under the metatarsal heads, or at the heel.

Typical causes of bursitis in the feet can be an injury or sustained pressure to a joint, or repetitive motions. Heel bursitis can manifest itself with the same symptoms as plantar fasciitis but the heel bursitis will persist with any weight-bearing activity whereas with plantar fasciitis the symptoms are relieved after the fascia warms up.

Treatments

The first action is to stop or reduce the motion or action that is causing the bursitis. The use of NSAIDS will help reduce the inflammation. Heat will relax the joint and promote tissue repair. In severe cases, fluid may be drawn from the sac to relieve pressure. Gently warming up before strenuous exercise can help avoid bursitis.

35

Numb Toes and Feet

The problem of numb feet can be one of two things either transient parasthesia or peripheral neuropathy. While each is bothersome, the first is usually temporary while the second can be very debilitating.

Transient Parasthesia

Transient parasthesia is a temporary nerve compression that can be caused by a gradual buildup of fluids in your feet during extended on-your-feet activity. As the feet swell and blood flow decreases, nerves become compressed. During the compression, the nerves do not receive the oxygen-rich blood they need, resulting in numbness and/or tingling. Tight shoes and/or tightly laced shoes contribute to the problem. Shoes with poor cushioning, coupled with a heavy, pounding gait can also may be a factor.

Ginny La Forma is an ultrarunner and adventure racer who has battled this numbness in her toes on many occasions. After the Hardrock 100-Mile Run, it lasted a few weeks, but after the Eco-Challenge it lasted over a year. She also suffers from Morton's Neuromas

If the problem continues after your activity has stopped, consider changing to more cushioned shoes, and changing insoles and arch supports. There may be some lymph system breakdown in the foot caused by micro-trauma. If the problem persist, consult a sports specialist.

Peripheral Neuropathy

Peripheral neuropathy is a painful nerve condition that can manifest itself as a burning sensation in the feet. It may start as a mild tingling in the toes and progress to searing pain. It can spread upward in the body, even to the thighs.

The pain results from damage to peripheral nerves that can come from a myriad of causes. A partial list of causes includes diabetes, kidney or liver disease, an underactive thyroid, viral and bacterial infections, vitamin deficiencies, pressure on a single nerve, although often, no cause is identified.

Symptoms include tingling, prickling, or numbness; the sensation of having an "invisible sock" on your feet; burning or freezing pain; a sharp, jabbing or electric type pain; extreme sensitivity to touch; muscle weakness; and a loss of balance or coordination.

A case study is shared by Ken Reed, an ultrarunner who discovered a year and one half ago that he had peripheral neuropathy. It started with a tingling in three of his left foot toes in the summer of '98 that later turned to numbness. That fall he sought medical advice when it progressed to shooting pains and aches. By spring of '99 it had progress to pains in his lower legs, with the numbness also moving upwards. Ken reports that when his feet are cold they constantly ache, buzz, and feel numb. He has resolved to managing the pain and discomfort, and hope for a miracle cure.

Treatments

Treatment often depends on the cause and symptoms of the neuropathy. It can be frustrating to treat, particularly if no reversible cause is identified. Typical treatments include pain relievers, either over-the-counter or prescribed for mild symptoms; tricyclic antidepressants for burning pain; antiseizure medications for jabbing pain; or other drugs.

Self-care treatments include proper care of your feet with loose socks and padded shoes; a semicircular hoop in bed to keep the cover off your feet; cold water soaks and skin moisturizers; massage to improve circulation and stimulate nerves; staying active; and reducing stress levels.

Products

Numb Toes and Aching Soles   This book is a must read for anyone experiencing peripheral neuropathy. Written by John A. Senneff, a peripheral neuropathy sufferer himself, the book deals with this disorder from the patient's perspective. Very well researched and readable. The ISBN to order the book is #096711017l8. It is available through bookstores, Healthy Legs & Feet Too! at www.healthy-legs.com or www.amazon.com.

Web Sites

Since peripheral neuropathy is so difficult to manage, the following web sites can offer some help.

- The Neuropathy Association – The online resource for peripheral neuropathy; www.neuropathy.org.
- Peripheral Neuropathy - The Neurological Disorder: www.neuropathy-trust.org.

36

Athlete's Foot

Athlete's foot, technically called *tinea pedis*, is a skin disease caused by a fungus. The hot weather and foot perspiration which athletes typically encounter can make athlete's foot a common problem. The combination of a warm and humid environment in the shoes or boots, excessive foot perspiration, and changes in the condition of the skin combine to create a setting for the fungi of athlete's foot to begin. Athlete's foot usually occurs between the toes or under the arch of the foot. Typical signs and symptoms of athlete's foot include itching, dry and cracking skin, inflammation with a burning sensation, and pain. Blisters and swelling may develop if left untreated. When these blisters break, small, red areas of raw tissue are exposed. As the infection spreads, the burning and itching will increase.

Aside from the cosmetic concerns toenail fungus can cause problems when the nail gets to thick. The solution is to keep it at a normal thickness. See the section *Toenail Problems* on page 224 for the proper technique to file nails.

Treatments

Treatment includes keeping the feet clean and dry, frequent socks changes, anti-fungal medications, and foot powders. The chapter *Powders* on page 79 has more information on choosing a foot powder. Anti-perspirants may also help those with excessive foot moisture. The chapter *Anti-Perspirants for the Feet* on page 129 has more information about these products. If you use a communal shower or bathroom after an event, or use a gym to train, avoid walking barefoot in these areas. Use thongs, shower booties, or even your shoes or boots.

Check your local drug store or pharmacy for a complete line of athlete's foot anti-fungal ointments, creams, liquids, powders, and sprays. See your doctor if your feet do not respond to treatment with over-the-counter medications.

Preventive measures include washing your feet daily with soap and water; drying them thoroughly, especially between the toes; wearing moisture-wicking socks; regularly changing your shoes and socks to control moisture; and the use of a good, moisture absorbing, foot powder.

If you have a fungal infection of the toenails, check with your local pharmacist for recommended medications. Use the medication as prescribed, for two to four weeks. If the fungus returns, alternate medications since it can sometimes build up a resistance to a particular fungicide. If it does not respond to treatment, a visit to your podiatrist may be necessary.

Products

Assorted Products   Check your local drug store and pharmacy for a current selection of related products. A sampling includes: Dr. Scholl's Fungal Nail Revitalizer, Dr. Scholl's Fungi Solution, Antifungal Lamisilat Cream, Lotrimin Antifungal AF Cream, Tinactin Antifungal Cream, Micatin Antifungal Cream, and Clotrimazole 1% Antifungal cream.

FootSmart   FootSmart carries Miracure Antifungal with 15% Aloe Vera and 1% Tolnaftate to rid the feet of Athlete's Foot and its itching. For information contact FootSmart Products, PO Box 922908, Norcross, GA 30010; (800) 870-7149; www.footsmart.com.

37

Plantar Warts

Plantar warts occasionally rear their ugly heads and cause foot pain. They can appear and then disappear suddenly, without any effort on your part, and may not recur for years. Usually painful from the pressure of standing and walking, plantar warts can become more painful due to running and hiking. These warts are typically small, hard, granulated lumps on the skin that can be flesh-colored, white, or pink. Warts are typically found on the bottom of the feet. Often a wart signals its presence feeling like a small stone is in your shoe. Most warts disappear without treatment in four to five months.

Plantar warts are benign tumors caused by common viral infections. They generally enter the sole of the foot through cuts and breaks in the skin. There are three types of warts. The first is a single, isolated wart. The second is one wart, often called the "mother," surrounded by any number of smaller "daughter" warts. The third type is a cluster of many warts grouped together, usually on the heels or the balls of the feet. Moist cracked skin and open or healing blisters leave one susceptible to the virus. To avoid getting a virus, do not walk barefoot in communal showers or bathrooms. Use thongs, shower booties, or even your shoes or boots.

Viruses cause warts. Viruses are

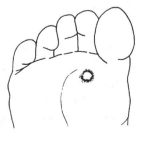

Plantar wart

living organisms and need oxygen. You can smother them by covering them with a piece of duct tape. The key is to keep it on as long as possible—usually several days—then replace it immediately when it gets loose. This is an effective way of getting rid of a wart. The problem is they tend to reoccur. The problem is that the body's immune system doesn't recognize them as invaders. Rich Schick, reports a study showed hypnotherapy to be effective in stimulating the immune system in curing warts, "As silly as it sounds a few minutes of concentrating on the area and thinking "wart go away" or "kill that wart" could be effective."

Treatments

While there are over-the-counter plantar wart removal compounds available, care must be taken in their use. Many products contain salicylic acid. Follow the product's directions to avoid damaging good tissue. Usually the treatment consists of applying the medication and covering the area with a bandage—repeating daily until the problem is resolved. Some individuals report success simply covering the wart with a piece of adhesive tape or even duct tape until the wart falls off. The common medical treatment by podiatrists for plantar warts involves the use of liquid nitrogen to freeze off the wart.

The treatments will put running or hiking on hold until after the spot heals, generally in about a week. Other treatment options include electrical burning, minor surgery, or laser surgery. Check with your podiatrist to determine your treatment options.

Products

Assorted Products   Check your local drug store and pharmacy for a current selection of related products. A sampling includes: Dr. Scholl's Clear-Away Plantar Wart Remover, Salicylic Acid Wart Remover Kit, DuoPlant Plantar Wart Remover, DuoFilm Patch System Wart Removal, and Wart-Off Wart Removal.

38

Cold & Heat Therapy

Cold therapy, sometimes referred to as cryotherapy, is an essential part of rehabilitation after an injury, as well as a prevention measure to avoid problems. Ice is usually done in combination with the other RICE components: Rest, Compression, and Elevation. Remember that all four are important and should be used together for faster recovery from an injury. Cold therapy can be used for sprains and strains, contusions and bruises, muscle pulls, and post exercise soreness.

The characteristics of icing move through four stages: cold, burning, aching, and finally numbness. The progression through the four stages usually takes about 20 minutes. The numbness stage should be reached in order to receive the full benefits of icing. The duration of icing depends on the type and depth of the injury. Body areas with less fat and tissue should be iced less that fatty or more dense areas (i.e., a bony area versus a hamstring). After an injury, soft tissue damage can cause uncontrolled swelling. This swelling can increase the damage of the initial injury and increase the healing time. The immediate use of ice will reduce the amount of swelling, tissue damage, blood clot formation, muscle spasms, inflammation, and pain. Ice also enhances the flow of nutrients to the injured area, which aids in the removal of waste products from the site and promotes healing.

Cold therapy works by constricting the blood vessels in the injured area and decreasing the tissue's temperature. The decreases blood flow, venous/lymphatic drainage, and cell metabolism, reducing the chance of hemorrhage and cell death in an acute injury. Once the fourth stage of icing, numbness, is reached, light range-of-motion can be started. Avoid strenuous exercise during cold therapy.

Do not place ice directly on the skin. Always use a thin towel, washcloth, or T-shirt between the ice bag and the skin. If you have an Ace wrap on the injured part, apply the ice directly over the wrap. Ice cubes in a Zip-Lock bag will work, but crushed ices conforms better to the body. When at home, a bag of frozen peas or corn also conforms nicely to the curves of the foot or ankle. Use an Ace wrap or other type compression wrap to hold the ice against the injured area. There are several recommendations regarding how long and how frequently to use ice.

- The typical recommendation is to apply ice three to four times daily to the injured area for 15 to 20 minutes at a time.
- Another recommendation is to ice for 20 minutes, wait ten minutes, and then reapply the ice for another 20 minutes. Repeat this three times a day for three days after an injury.

Ice massage can be done by freezing water in a paper or foam cup. When frozen, remove part of the cup and rub the ice around the injured area. Because it cools the area faster than normal icing, limit the massage to six to eight minutes at a time, usually three to four times a day. Ice massage is effective when used with range-of-motion exercises and stretching.

Heat therapy is used less often than cold therapy. Heat therapy is recommended only after swelling and inflammation have sub-sided (usually at least 72 hours after an injury). The heat increases blood flow to the injured area. The blood's nutrients help in the healing process. Heat can help reduce muscle spasms and reduce pain. Stiffness is decreased and tissue elasticity is increased. Heat should not be applied for longer than 15-20 minutes at a time.

Do not use cold or heat therapy on an area where the skin is broken. First treat the wound. Individuals with known or suspected circulatory problems or cold hypersensitivity, paralysis or areas of impaired sensation, or rheumatoid conditions should consult a physician before using cold compression therapy.

Products

Contour Pak   The Contour Pak Cold Flex Wrap is an all-purpose cold therapy wrap that contours to the foot and ankle as well and other parts of the body: knee, hamstring, neck, shoulder, lower back, etc. This unique wrap uses a non-toxic gel formulation that never freezes solid so it stays soft and flexible while cold, retaining its therapeutic temperatures for 30 to 40 minutes. It has a soft, velvety fabric covering that eliminates the need to use a towel between the pack and the skin and protects against ice burn. Elastic straps with Velcro are used to hold the wrap snuggly in place over the desired body part. For more information contact Contour Pak, PO Box 162, Moraga, CA 94556; (800) 926-2228; www.hooked.net/~contour.

DuckPads Basic Web   Tikoor makes DuckPads' Basic Web packs to be used either chilled or heated. Their sandal-like design fits around the foot. They contain a non-toxic gel that works well whether chilled or heated. The gel is on the bottom and up the sides of the ankle and forefoot. The Basic Web comes in men's and women's sizes based on your shoe size. For more information contact Tikoor, 9000 Crow Canyon Road, Danville, CA 94506; (877) 4DUCKPD; www.tikoor.com.

Homemade Ice Pack   A homemade ice bag can be made with three parts water and one part rubbing alcohol. Mix in a heavy-duty Zip-Lock bag and keep one or two in the freezer. What this combination makes is a hard slush. If the mix is too hard, let it melt and add a little more alcohol. If it is too liquid, add a little more water. The right consistency will allow the bag to be formed around your foot, ankle, or other body part. Use a towel between the ice bag and your skin.

Solar Polar Hot / Cold Therapy Packs   Thermal Logic makes hot and cold packs with a unique cross-linked polymer gel that stays soft and pliable even below freezing. Heat and cold is retained for hours. This gel is not a liquid so there is no dander of leakage if the pack is punctured. A contoured Ankle Pack is available that uses elastic and Velcro straps to form a snug fit. Other sizes are offered. It can be stored in the freezer or place it in the microwave to use as a heat pack. For more information contact Thermal Logic, 9300 Industrial Drive, Bastrop, LA 71220; (800) 385-9544; www.thermal-logic.com.

39

Foot Care Kits

There are two types of kits. The first is a basic self-care kit for keeping your feet healthy and the second is to carry with you in the field or wherever your sport takes you. Each is equally important.

A basic self-care kit for good foot treatment does not have to be large. The following items are basic. Add to the kit as necessary for your particular foot conditions.

- Toenail clippers to trim nails
- File or emery board to smooth nails after clipping
- Foot powder to absorb moisture
- Moisturizer crème to soften dry skin and calluses and corns
- Pumice stone to remove calluses and dead skin
- Antiseptic ointment for cuts, scrapes

If you are an athlete who finds yourself continuously bothered by foot problems, or who often covers long distances without crew support, consider making a small foot care kit to carry in a fanny pack. Hikers should carry a kit, as part of a larger overall first-aid kit, because of their remoteness from assistance. The following items are recommended.

- Tincture of benzoin swabsticks or squeeze vials
- Alcohol wipe packets
- A nail clippers or pin, and matches for blister puncturing

- Foot powder in a 35mm film canister (with a salt shaker top found at backpacking stores)
- A small container for your choice of a lubricant
- Your choice of tapes wrapped around a pencil
- A plastic bag with your choice of blister materials and several pieces of toilet paper or tissues
- A small pocket knife with a built-in scissors

You may consider other options to include in the kit, based on your personal foot problems or injury history.

- A lightweight ankle support
- Pads for metatarsal, arch, or heel pain
- A heel cup

You can make your own blister kit as described above or purchase a general first-aid kit or a blister medical kit. Most general first-aid kits contain items for basic first-aid care and can be used for blister care by adding a few more specific items. The kits mentioned below are made specifically for blister care. No matter what each kit contains, you should customize the kit to suit your needs and stock it with sufficient equipment for your outing.

Products

Brave Soldier Wound Healing Ointment This ointment was made for athletes and is popular among bicyclists. Developed by a dermatologist as an effective treatment to keep abrasion wounds moist and protected, Brave Soldier helps heal blisters, road rash, minor cuts and burns. Made with tea tree oil as a natural antiseptic, aloe gel for its natural healing properties, jojoba oil as a natural moisturizer, Vitamin E to rebuild collagen and skin tissue, shark liver oil to reduce scarring, and comfrey to stimulate skin cell growth and wound resurfacing. For more information contact Brave Soldier, 8330 Beverly Blvd., Los Angeles, CA 90048; (888) 711-BRAV; www.bravesoldier.com.

Blister Fighter Medical Kit Outdoor Research offers

an 11-ounce Blister Fighter Medical Kit which can be carried in a backpack or kept in a gear bag. The kit contains moleskin, tape, bandages, 2nd Skin pads, Poron donuts, bandage scissors, a razor blade, needles, antibacterial towelettes, iodine and lidocaine wipes, benzoin, antibiotic ointment, foot powder, a zip-top bag, and a *Blister Fighter Guide* booklet. The kit comes in a zippered nylon pouch. For more information contact Outdoor Research, 2203 1st Avenue South, Seattle, WA 98134-1424; (888) 4OR-GEAR; www.orgear.com. Sold only through distributors, no online sales.

Blister Resister Medical Kit   This second kit by Outdoor Research offers a 7 ½-ounce smaller version of the Blister Fighter Medical Kit. The kit has less of everything and does not include the scissors, lidocaine wipes, and foot powder. Contact Outdoor Research as noted above.

Cramer Blister Kit   The Cramer Blister Kit comes with five soft, super thin, adhesive-backed foam pads and five alcohol prep pads. For more information contact Cramer Products, Inc. PO Box 1001, Gardner, KS 66030; (800) 255-6621; www.cramersportsmed.com. Available through distributors or from Medco Sports Medicine (see page 273).

Mueller Blister Kit   This blister kit contains three hydrogel pads, three providone-iodine wipes, and mesh tape for securing the pads. Look for this kit in backpacking or sporting goods stores or contact Mueller Sports Medicine, Inc., One Quench Drive, Prairie du Sac, WI 53578; (800) 356-9522; www.muellersportsmed.com. Available through distributors or from Medco Sports Medicine (see page 273).

Spenco Blister Kit   This blister kit contains six 2nd Skin 1″ squares, six sheets of Adhesive Knit, and one sheet of Pressure Pad ovals. The kit comes in a resealable pouch. Look for this kit in backpacking or sporting goods stores or contact Spenco Medical Corporation, PO Box 2501, Waco, TX 76702-2501; (800) 877-3626; www.spenco.com.

Part Four

Sources and Resources

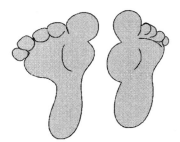

40

Medical and Footwear Specialists

American Academy of Podiatric Sports Medicine
1729 Glastonberry Road
Potomac, MD 20854
(800) 438-3355
www.aapsm.org
Referrals for podiatrists

American Chiropractors Association
(800) 986-4636
www.americhiro.org

American Academy of Orthopaedic Surgeons
(800) 346-AAOS
www.aaos.org
Referrals for orthopedic surgeons

American Massage Therapy Association
(847) 864-0123
www.amtamassage.org

American Orthopaedic Foot and Ankle Society
1216 Pine Street, Suite 201
Seattle, WA 98101
(800) 235-4855
www.aofas.org

American Orthotics and Prosthetics Association
1650 King Street, Suite 500
Alexandria, VA 22314
(703) 836-7116
www.aopanet.org

American Physical Therapy Association
(800) 999-2782
www.apta.org

American Podiatric Medical Association
9312 Old Georgetown Road
Bethesda, MD 20814-1698
(800) FOOTCARE
www.apma.org

International Chiropractic Association
(800) 423-4690
www.chiropractic.org

National Athletic Trainers' Association
(800) 879-6282
www.nata.org

Pedorthic Footwear Association
9861 Broken Land Parkway, Suite 255, Columbia, MD 21046-1151
(800) 673-8447
www.pedorthics.org

41

Shoe Review and Gear Review Sources

Adventure World Magazine
PO Box 20113
San Jose, CA 95160
(408) 997-3581
www.csmevents.com
Articles on adventure racing, including multi-day events.
Occasional gear reviews and training articles.

Backpacker Magazine
Rodale Press, Inc., 33 E. Minor Street, Emmaus, PA 18098
Customer Service Department: (800) 666-3434
www.bpbasecamp.com
The March issue is their Annual Gear Guide which reviews
footwear.

Marathon & Beyond Magazine
42K(+) Press, Inc.
411 Park Lane Drive
Champaign, IL 61820
(217) 359-9345
www.marathonandbeyond.com
Occasional articles on sports injuries and fitness.

Outside Magazine
400 Market St., Santa Fe, NM 87501

Customer Service Department: (800) 678-1131
www.outsidemag.com
The Buyer's Guide is a special magazine typically issued in
May.

Runner's World Magazine
Rodale Press, Inc., 33 E. Minor Street, Emmaus, PA 18098
Customer Service Department: (800) 666-2828
www.runnersworld.com
The April (Spring), and October (Fall), and December (Winter)
issues usually have shoe reviews.

Running Times Magazine
Fitness Publishing, Inc., 98 N. Washington St., Boston, MA
02114
Subscriptions and inquiries: (800) 816-4735
The March (Spring) and September (Fall) issues usually have
shoe reviews.

Trail Runner Magazine
North South Publications, Inc., 603 South Broadway, Suite A,
Boulder, CO 80303
(303) 499-8410
www.trailrunnermag.com
The Spring and Fall issues usually have shoe reviews.

UltraRunning Magazine
PO Box 2120
Amherst, MA 01004-2120
(413) 584-2640
www.ultrarunning.com
Occasional gear reviews and articles with personal experiences
and tips.

42

Internet Feet-Related Web Sites

Barefoot Dirty Sole Society
www.barefooters.org

Footcare Direct – Foot, Ankle and Heel Information.
www.footcaredirect.com/index.html#index

Foot Express: Footcare Home Health Products and Treatments
www.footexpress.com

Foot Web: Footcare Treatment Information Resource
www.footweb.com

Healthy Legs & Feet Too!: Promoting Leg and Foot Health
www.healthy-legs.com

LaFoot Plus: A Sports Health & Wellness Center
www.lafoot.com

Podiatry links
www.footandankle.com/podmed

Running Barefoot
www.barefoot.cecs.csulb.edu/running

The Ambulatory Foot Clinic - Podiatric Pain Management Center
www.footcare4u.com

The Foot Store – Products for foot support and comfort by certified pedorthists
www.footstore.com

Walking information
www.walking.about.com/sports/walking

43

Product Sources

When products are mentioned in the text, the company name, address, telephone number, and Internet web site (if available), are provided. Some companies may not sell retail but should be able to identify a local distributor. Generally, your first source for most of these products should be your local stores. Ask at your running store, backpacking or camping store, pharmacy or drug store, medical supply store, or orthopedic supply store for the products mentioned. While they may not stock all the products mentioned, they may be willing to place a special order.

Medco Sports Medicine is a distributor that offers many of the products mentioned in this book through their Internet web site and catalogue. Some individuals will find them a convenient source.

- **Medco Sports Medicine**, 500 Fillmore Avenue, Tonawanda, NY 14150; (800) 556-3326 (24-hours a day); www.medco.com.
  Medco carries tapes; self-adhering wraps; tape adherents and skin tougheners; various grades of moleskin; lubricants, powders, first-aid equipment; alcohol and tincture of benzion prep pads; anti-fungal sprays and powders; hot and cold therapy equipment; physical therapy equipment; ankle supports; Achilles tendon and plantar fasciitis straps; insoles and heel cups (including Bauerfeind Viscoelastic insoles); most Cramer, Mueller and Spenco products; and Johnson &

Johnson Band-Aid Blister Relief, Corn Relief, and Callus Relief.

You may find products similar to those mentioned which are only available in your area. Watching other athletes will often lead to new products they have found to be useful in their foot care efforts. Do not hesitate to ask questions when you see new products.

Rather than use this book as a definitive source, use it as a guide to the wide variety of foot care products available. New products are always being developed. Remember too, your local stores are an excellent source for what is current in the foot care marketplace.

Please be aware that not all companies sell retail and therefore their products may have to be ordered through a store, pharmacy or drug store, podiatrist or orthopedist, or a medical supply or orthopedic supply dealer. Please respect their sales policies.

Glossary

Achilles Tendon The large tendon which runs from the calf to the back of the heel.

Adventure Racing Multi-sport races over difficult terrain, often done in teams over several days.

Arch The curved part of the bottom of the foot.

Athlete's Foot Itchy, red, soggy, flaking and cracking skin between the toes or fluid-filled bumps on the sides or sole of the foot caused by a fungal infection.

Biomechanics The study of the mechanics of a living body, especially of the forces exerted by muscles and gravity on the skeletal structure.

Blister A sac between layer of skin filled with fluid that occurs as a result of friction.

Bone Spur A small bony growth usually indicating a bone irritation.

Bruise An injury in which blood vessels beneath the skin are broken and blood escapes to produce a discolored area.

Bunion A bony protrusion at the base of the big toe.

Bunionette A bunion on the small toe.

Calcaneous The large heel bone.

Calluses The thickening of skin caused by recurring friction, usually on the sole of the foot, the heel, or the inner big toe.

Contusion A bruising injury that does not involve a break in the skin.

Corns Thickening of the skin, generally on or between the toes, usually caused by friction.

Dermis The sensitive connective tissue layer of the skin located below the epidermis, containing nerve endings, sweat and sebaceous glands, and blood and lymph vessels.

Dislocation A complete displacement of bone from its normal position at the joint surface

Edema The swelling of body tissues due to excessive fluid.

Epidermis The outer, protective, nonvascular layer of the skin covering the dermis.

Eversion Movement of the outside of the foot upward as the foot rolls to the inside.

Fibula The outer and smaller of the two bones of the lower leg.

Flat Foot A foot that has either a low arch or no arch.

Forefoot The ball of the foot and the toes.

Heel Pad The soft tissue pad on the bottom of the heel.

Heel Spur A small edge of bone which juts out of the calcaneous.

Hematoma A swelling that contains blood beneath the skin due to an injury to a blood vessel.

Hot Spot A hot and reddened area of skin that has been irritated by friction.

Hyperhidrosis Excessive moisture.

Infection Condition in which a part of the body is invaded by a microorganism such as a bacteria or virus.

Inversion Movement of the inside of the foot upward as the foot rolls to the outside.

Last The form over which a shoe or boot is constructed.

Lateral The outside of the foot, leg, or body.

Ligaments The strong fibrous connective tissue at a joint that connects one bone to another bone.

Maceration A breaking down or softening of skin tissue by extended exposure to moisture.

Medial The inside of the foot, legs, or body.

Metatarsalgia Pain somewhere underneath the metatarsal heads of the foot.

Midfoot The mid or center part of the foot containing the arch and five metatarsal bones.

Morton's Neuroma Pain on the bottom of the foot, usually under the pad of the third or fourth toe.

Morton's Foot A foot type where the second toe is longer than the big toe.

Neuroma The swelling of a nerve due to an inflammation of the nerve or the tissue surrounding the nerve.

Orthopedist An orthopedic surgeon specializing in the treatment and surgery of bones and joint injuries, diseases, and problems.

Orthotics A molded insert made from a mold of the bottom of the foot which is then inserted into a shoe or boot to correct a foot abnormality.

Pedorthist A specialist trained to work on the fit or modification of shoes and orthotics to alleviate foot problems caused by disease, overuse, or injury.

Plantar Fascia The band of fibers along the arch of the foot which connects the heel to the toes.

Plantar Fasciitis An inflammation of the plantar fascia.

Plantar Warts Small, hard, flesh colored, white, or pink granulated lumps typically found on the feet and caused by a virus.

Podiatrist A doctor of podiatric medicine who specializes in the treatment and surgery of the foot and ankle.

Pronation An abnormal rolling over of the foot towards the inside of the body when weight bearing.

RICE The acronym for rest, ice, compression and elevation, which are used for sprain and strain injuries.

Sesamoiditis An inflammation of the two little bones beneath the ball of the foot, under the joint that moves the big toe.

Sole The bottom of the foot.

Sprain A joint injury in which ligament damage is sustained.

Sterilization The process of the removal of bacteria.

Strain   Muscular injury produced by overuse or abuse of a muscle.

Subluxation   An incomplete or partial dislocation.

Subungal Hematoma   A hemotoma under the nail plate.

Supination   The rolling of the foot towards the outside of the body when weight bearing.

Tendinitis   An inflammation of a tendon or its surrounding sheath.

Tendons   The elastic tough fibrous tissue that connects muscles to bone.

Toe Box   The front part of a shoe or boot that covers the toes.

Ultrarunning   Running distances greater than a marathon.

Virus   A tiny organism that causes disease.

Wart   A thickened, painful area of skin caused by a virus.

Endnotes

[1] Roland Mueser, *Long-Distance Hiking: Lessons from the Appalachian Trail* (Camden, Maine: Rugged Mountain Press, 1998), p. 32.

[2] J.J. Knapik, K.I. Reynolds, K.L. Duplantis, and B.H. Jones. "Friction Blisters: Pathophysiology, Prevention and Treatment." *Sports Medicine* (20 (3) 1995), p. 140.

[3] 12 miles per day times, 5,280 feet/mile divided by 2.5 feet/step. For each mile more than 12 add 2100 steps. For each mile less than 12 subtract 2100 steps.

[4] Ray Jardine, *The Pacific Crest Trail Hiker's Handbook* (LaPine, OR: Adventure Lore Press, 1996), p. 93.

[5] Karen Berger, *Advanced Backpacking* (New York, NY: W.W. Norton & Company, 1998), p. 69-70.

[6] The usual issues are: *Backpacking* (March is the Annual Gear Guide Issue), *Outside* (May Buyer's Guide), *Runner's World* (April and September), *Running Times* (March and September) and *Trail Runner* (Spring and Fall).

[7] J.D. Denton, Dennis Grandy, D.P.M., and Tom Kennedy, "How to Find the Right Shoe for You" *Running Times* (September 1996), p. 16, and "How to Find a Shoe That Works." *Running Times* (March 1997), p. 18.

[8] Tom Brunick, and Bob Wischnia, "Choosing the Right Shoe" and "Know Your Foot Type." *Runner's World* (April 1997), p. 52.

[9] J.J. Knapik, K.L. Reynolds, K.L. Duplantis, and B.H. Jones,

"Friction Blisters: Pathophysiology, Prevention, and Treatment." *Sports Medicine* (20 (3) 1995), p. 142.

[10]   Tim Noakes, MD, *The Lore of Running* (Champaign, IL: Leisure Press, 1991), p. 460.

[11]   Robert Boeder, *Beyond the Marathon: The Grand Slam of Trail   Ultrarunning* (Vienna, GA: Old Mountain Press, 1996), p. 22.

[12]   J.J. Knapik, K.L. Reynolds, K.L. Duplantis, and B.H. Jones, "Friction Blisters: Pathophysiology, Prevention and Treatment." *Sports Medicine* (20 (3) 1995), p. 139.

[13]   Andrew Lovy, "New Blister Formula Revealed! Free!" *UltraRunning* (April 1990), p. 40.

[14]   Colin Fletcher, *The Complete Walker III* (New York: Alfred A. Knopf, 1996), p. 86.

[15]   Richard Benyo, *The Death Valley 300: Near-Death and Resurrection on the World's Toughest Endurance Course* (Forestville: Specific Publications, 1991), p. 142.

[16]   Gary Cantrell, "From the South: The Amazing Miracle of Duct Tape." *UltraRunning* (December, 1988), p. 36-37.

[17]   Donald Baxter, MD; David Porter, MD, Ph.D.; Paul Flahavan, C.Ped; and Charles May, "The Ideal Running Orthosis: A Philosophy of Design." *Biomechanics* (March, 1996), p. 41-44.

[18]   Tim Noakes, MD, *The Lore of Running* (Champaign, IL: Leisure Press, 1991), p. 459.

[19]   J.J. Knapik, K.L. Reynolds, K.L. Duplantis, and B.H. Jones, "Friction Blisters: Pathophysiology, Prevention and Treatment." *Sports Medicine* (20 (3) 1995), p. 138.

[20]   Ibid., p. 140.

[21]   Ibid., p. 139.

[22]   Bryan Bergeron, MD, "A Guide to Blister Management." *The Physician and Sportsmedicine* (February 1995), p. 40.

[23]   Ibid., p. 43.

[24]   William Trolan, MD, *Blister Fighter Guide* (Seattle: Outdoor Research 1996).

[25]   Auleley, Guy-Robert, MD, et al. "Valudation of the Ottowa Ankle Rules" Annals of Emergency Medicine: 32(1); 14-18.

July 1998.

[26] "The Conservative Treatment of Plantar Fasciitis; A Prospective Randomized, Multicenter Outcome Study" (American Orthopaedic Foot and Ankle Society, October 1996).

[27] Robert Nirschl, MD. MS, "Plantar Fasciitis — A New Perspective." *American Medical Joggers Association AMAA Quarterly.* (Summer 1996).

[28] Karen Maloney Backstrom, C. Forsyth, B. Walden, Abstract: Comparison of Two Methods of Stretching the Gastrocnemius and Their Effects on Ankle Range of Motion." University of Colorado Health Services Center, Denver, CO, April, 1994.

Bibliography

Ellis, Joe, D.P.M. with Joe Henderson. *Running Injury-Free*. Emmaus, PA: Rodale Press, 1994.

Jardine, Ray. *The Pacific Crest Trail Hiker's Handbook*. LaPine, OR: AdventureLore Press, 1996.

Levine, Suzanne M., MD. *My Feet are Killing Me!* New York: McGraw-Hill Book Company, 1987.

McGann Daniel M, D.P.M. and L. R. Robinson. *The Doctor's Sore Foot Book*. New York: William Morrow and Company, Inc., 1991.

Noakes, Tim, MD. *The Lore of Running*. Champaign, IL: Leisure Press, 1991.

Salmans, Sandra. *Your Feet: Questions you have ... Answers you need*. Allentown, PA: People's Medical Society, 1998.

Schneider, Myles J., D.P.M. and Mark D. Sussman, D.P.M. *How to Doctor Your Feet Without a Doctor*. Washington, D.C.: Acropolis Books, Ltd., 1984.

Subotnick, Steven I., D.P.M., M.S. *The Running Foot Doctor*. San Francisco: World Publications, 1977.

——, *Sports & Exercise Injuries: Conventional, Homeopathic, & Alternative Treatments*. Berkeley: North Atlantic Books, 1991.

Tremain, David M., MD and Elias M. Awad, Ph.D. *The Foot & Ankle Sourcebook*. Los Angeles: Lowell House, 1996.

Taliaferro Blauvelt, Carolyn and Nelson, Fred R.T. *A Manual of Orthopaedic Terminology*, Fifth Edition. St. Louis: Mosby Year Books, 1994.

Trolan, William, MD. *Blister Fighter Guide*. Seattle: Outdoor Research, 1996.

Weisenfeld, Murry F., MD with Barbara Burr. *The Runner's Repair Manual*. New York: St. Martin's Press, 1980.

About the Author

John Vonhof brings a varied background and extensive experience to *Fixing Your Feet*. This second edition, which he wrote and illustrated, is the synthesis of over 20 years of experience as a runner and hiker.

Having run since 1982, John discovered the challenging world of trail running and ultras in 1984. Over the years, he has completed more than 20 ultras: 50Ks, 50-milers, 100-milers, 24-hour runs, and a 72-hour run. John has completed the difficult Western States 100 Mile Endurance Run three times and the Santa Rosa 24-Hour and 12-Hour Track Runs 12 times.

In 1987 John, with fellow runner Will Uher, fastpacked the 211-mile John Muir Trail in the California High Sierra's in 8.5 days with 30 pound packs. Other summers have been spent doing other Sierra backpacks.

As race director of the Ohlone Wilderness 50 KM Trail Run for the past 13 years, John has worked at providing a quality event for runners of all skill levels. This run is known as one of the most difficult 50-KM trail ultras in Northern California.

An opportunity to change careers in 1992 led him into the medical field where he now works as an emergency room/trauma technician with certifications as a paramedic and orthopedic technician. Over the years he has provided volunteer medical aid at numerous running events.

This background has provided a wealth of learning opportunities for what can go wrong with feet and ways to fix them.

Index

A

Accommodator Orthotics 204, 213
Achilles tendinitis 217
Achilles Tendon Strap 221
Acorn Fleece Socks 69, 75
Adhesive felt 172
Advanced blister care 173
Adventure racing 14
Adventure World Magazine 269
Air-Lace Shoelaces 142
Alignment, of the body 20
American Academy of Orthopaedic Surgeons 9, 42, 267
American Academy of Podiatric Sports Medicine 267
American Chiropractors Association 267
American Massage Therapy Association 267
American Orthopaedic Foot and Ankle Society 9, 267
American Orthotics and Prosthetics Association 268
American Physical Therapy Association 268
American Podiatric Medical Association 268
Anatomy of Footwear 28
Andrew Lovy's lubricant formula 82
Ankle supports 191
Anti-Perspirants for the Feet 129
Arch, of the foot 20
Arch Crafters Custom-Fit Insoles 47, 118
Asphalt, running on 23
Athletes foot 253

Athletic trainers 10
Avon
  Double Action Foot File 245
  Silicone Glove lubricant 82

B

Backpacker Magazine 269
Bag Balm lubricant 82
Barefoot Dirty Sole Society 271
Barefoot hiking 76
Barefoot running 76
Basic blister repair 169
BaySix socks 66
Betadine 89, 122
Bio Skin 192
Biomechanical problems 20
Biomechanically efficient 40
Biomechanics 19
Blister Fighter Medical Kit 262
Blister Guard technology 63
Blister prevention components 56
Blister Relief 174
Blister Resister Medical Kit 263
Blisters 163
  advanced blister care 173
  beyond blisters 182
  blister development 15, 164
  blisters, factors which cause 55
  blood-filled blisters 171
  changing insoles to avoid 45
  dehydration, in causing 125
  draining the blister 169
  extreme blister prevention and care 177
  foot changes, with blister care products 183
  four therapeutic goals of blister management 168
  friction, in blister development 165
  from bad fitting footwear 42
  general blister care 168
  infected blisters 171, 172
  moisture, in causing 55
  ruptured blisters 171

sterile wound dressings 182
Blisters, basics of 164
BodyGlide lubricant 83
Brave Soldier Wound Healing Ointment 172, 262
Bridgedale socks 69, 75
Bromi-Talc powder 80
Buddy taping 223
Bunion and bunionettes 246
Bursitis 248
Buying shoes 42

C

Callus Treatment Cream 123, 245
Calluses 121, 242
Changing your shoes and socks 145
Chiropractors 11
Cho-Pat
    Achilles Tendon Strap 221
    Ankle Support 192
Chondroitin sulfate 189
Chronic foot problems 11
Coban 177, 182
Cold therapy 257
Compeed 174
Components of prevention 55
Conditioning, of the feet 17
Corns 241
Cornstarch 79
Count'R-Force Arch Brace 204, 213
Cramer
    Blister Kit 263
    Heel Cup 204
    Tuf-Skin 88
Crew Support 149
Cropper Medical Bio Skin 192
Custom orthotic alternatives 117
Custom-made orthotics 116
Customizing your footwear 44

D

Dahlgren socks 69
Dehydration 125, 147
Demands on your feet 13
Dermis 165
Dislocations 198
Double-layer socks 64
Downhill, running 24
Draining the blister 169
DRYZ Insoles 47, 131
DuckPads Basic Web 259
Duct tape techniques 94

E

E-CAPS Endurolytes 126
Easy Laces 143
Electrolytes 125
Epidermis 165
Extreme blister prevention and care 177
    Instant Krazy Glue 180
    New Skin Liquid Bandage 180
    tincture of benzoin and silicone cream 178
    tincture of benzoin inside a blister 179
    using tape 178

F

Fit
    factors affecting 27
    getting a proper fit 38
Flat-arched feet 41
Foot bones 19
    metatarsal bones 20
Foot care kits 261, 263
Foot Express 271
Foot Solution 131
Foot Solution anti-perspirant 131
Foot types 40
Foot Web 271
Footcare Direct 271

FootSmart 122, 227, 231, 234, 236, 242, 245, 247, 254
Fox River socks 66, 69, 71
Fractures 194
Friction, cause of blisters 55, 165
Frostbite 146

G

Gaiters 133
  homemade gaiters 135
  role in preventing blisters 133
Getting a proper fit 38
Glucosamine sulfate 189
Gold Bond powder 80, 131
Gordons #5 anti-perspirant 132

H

Hammer toes 230
Hapad
  Arch Pads 214
  Comf-Orthotic 47, 119
  Heel Pads and Cushions 204, 221
  Insoles 47
  Metatarsal Pads and Bars 234, 236, 238, 242, 245, 247
  Tongue Cushion 143
Healthy Legs & Feet Too! 271
Heat
  cause of blisters 55
  for injuries 189
Heat therapy 258
Heel Bed 4pf 205
Heel Hugger 205
Heel problems
  heel and arch discomfort 202
  heel cups and pads 202
  heel neuromas 202
  heel pain 21
  nerve entrapment syndromes 202
  plantar fasciitis, related to heel pain 202
  stretching, to resolve heel pain 203
Heel spurs 201

Helly-Hansen socks　71
Hhyponatremia　125
High-arched feet　41
High-technology oversocks　72
Hiking　13
Hiking boots　33
　　flexion　36
　　weight of　35
Hiking socks　68
Homemade gaiters　135
Homemade ice pack　259
Hot spots　161
Hydration　125
Hydropel lubricant　83

I

Ice massage　189, 258
Ingrown toenails　224
Injury　9, 21
Insoles　45
International Chiropractic Association　268
Internet Feet-Related Web Sites　271
Blister management　168

K

Kallassy Ankle Support　192
Krazy Glue　180

L

Lacing options　139
LaFoot Plus　271
Lanolin cream　83
Last, of shoe construction　29
Ligaments　19
　　nutritional supplements for healing　189, 219
Longitudinal arches　20
Lubricants　81
Lynco Biomechanical Orthotic Systems　119, 205, 214

M

Marathon & Beyond Magazine 269
Massage 122
Massage therapists 11
Medco Sports Medicine 273
Medical and footwear specialists 9, 267
MetaPumper Orthotics 118
Metatarsalgia 233
MiniGators 136
Moisture, cause of blisters 55
Moleskin 169, 172, 181
Morton's Foot 229
Mortons neuroma 235
Mueller
    Blister Kit 263
    More Skin 175
    Tuffner Clear Spray 88
Multi-Day Events 153

N

National Athletic Trainers' Association 268
Nerve compression 249
Nerve inflammation 235
Neuropathy Association 251
New Skin Liquid Bandage 88, 175, 180
N'ice Stretch Night Splint Suspension System 214, 221
Normal arched feet 41
Not wearing socks 76
NSAIDS inflammatories 187
Numb toes and feet 249
Nutrition for the feet 121
Nutritional supplements, for healing 189, 219

O

Odor-Eater's Foot Powder 80
Orthopedists 9
Orthotics 115
Ottowa Ankle Rules 195
Outdoor Research gaiters 136
Outside Magazine 269

P

Pain
    foot pain 11
    heel pain 201
    recurring pain 9
Patagonia socks 70, 71
Pedorthic Footwear Association 268
Pedorthists 10, 44
Perform 8 Lateral Ankle Stabilizer 193
Peripheral Neuropathy 250
Persistent foot problems 9
Perspiration 129
PF Night Splint 214
Physical therapists 10
Plantar fasciitis 209
    arch brace 211
    night splint 211, 219
    stretching 210
    treatments 210
Plantar reFLEX Night Splint 215, 222
Plantar warts 255
Podiatrists 9
Podiatry links 271
Powders 79
Powerstep Insoles 205, 215
Preventive maintenance 3, 53
Preventing infection 171
Prevention 53
Proactive 3, 53
Product sources 273
Pronation 21, 40
ProStretch 206, 215, 222
PSC - Pronation/Spring Control 206, 215

R

RaceReady Trail Gaitors 136
Reactive 3, 53
REI Socks 70
REI/Gore-Tex Oversocks 73
Repairing gaiter straps 134

RICE, treatment for sprains and strains 186, 218
Ridgeview socks 66
Roads, running on 23
Rubbing alcohol 88
Runique socks 66
Runner's Lube lubricant 83
Runners' World Magazine *270*
Running barefoot 271
Running shoes 29
   for hiking 36
   last, of shoe construction 29
Running socks 65
Running Times Magazine *270*

S

Sandal socks 75
Sandals 37
SealSkinz Waterproof MVT Socks 73
Second Wind Insoles 47
Seirus Neo-Sock and StormSock 74
Selecting hiking boots 34
Self-adherent wrap 177
Sesamoiditis 237
Shoe review and gear review sources 269
Sidewalks, running on 23
Skin tougheners 87
Skin-Lube lubricant 84
SmartWool socks 66, 70, 71
Sock liners 71
Socks 61
   double-layer socks 64
   fitting socks 64
   high-technology oversocks 72
   hiking socks 68
   running socks 65
   sandal socks 75
   sock liners 71
   the option of not wearing socks 76
   types of socks 62
Sodium 125
Sof Sole Insoles 47

Solar Polar Hot / Cold Therapy Packs 259
Spectrum Sports Insoles 48
Spenco 48
 2nd Skin 176
 Cushions 234, 237, 238
 Adhesive Knit 176
 Blister Kit 263
 Iinsoles 48
 Multi-Fresh socks 66, 70
 Orthotic Arch Support 120
 Pressure Pads 173
Sport Similarities 14
Sport Slick lubricant 84
Sports and and your feet 13
Sports medicine doctors 10
SportSlick lubricant 84
Sportsloob lubricant 84
Sprains 185
 ankle supports 191
Spur Relief Heel Cup 206
Spyroflex 176
Sterile wound dressings, for blisters 182
Strains 185
 ankle supports 191
Strassburg Sock 206, 216, 222
Strengthening exercises, for sprains and strains 189
Stress Fractures 196
Stromgren Ankle Support 193
Stubbed toes 223, 227
Subungal hematoma 225
SUCCEED! Buffer/Electrolyte Caps 126
Superfeet Insoles 48
Supination 21, 40
Suzi's Taping Techniques 97
Syringes and Needles 179, 181

T

TacLiner Insoles 48
TacTape 49, 120
TakeOff Ankle Protec Wrap 193
Tape adherents 87

Taping
  applying the tape 92
  basics 91
  duct tape techniques 94
  finishing touches 93
  preparing the skin 92
  removing tape 93
  Suzi taping technique 97
  tape adherents 91, 92
  taping basics 91
  taping between toe and foot 96
  taping over blisters 93
  taping the ball of the foot 95
  taping the bottom of the foot 98
  taping the bottom of the heel 97
  taping the sides of the foot 98
  taping the toes 96, 99
  types of tape 91
Tea and Betadine skin toughener 89
Teamwork, and footcare 149
Tendons 19
  nutritional supplements, for healing 189, 219
Terrain 23
The Ambulatory Foot Clinic 272
The Foot Store 272
The Ultimate Heel & Arch Support 207, 216
Thermohair socks 70, 75
Thermotabs 126
Thorlo socks 67, 70
Tincture of benzoin 89, 92, 173
Tired feet 160
Toenail problems
  black toenail 225
  ingrown toenails 224
  toenail fungus 225
Tom Crawford's tea and Betadine skin toughener 89
Total Foot Recovery Cream 123, 245
Tracks, running on 25
Trails, running on 24
Training 54
Transient parasthesia 249

Transverse arch 20
Treatment, seeking medical 3
Treatments, to fix your feet 159
Types of socks 62

U

Udder Balm 84
Ultrarunning Magazine *13*
Un-Petroleum Jelly lubricant 85
Uphill running 24
Using syringes and needles 181

V

Vaseline 85
Viruses 255
Viscoheel 207
Viscoped 235, 237, 239
Viscoped S 216

W

Walking information 272
Ways to prevent blisters 101
Weight of your shoes/boots 35
Western States 100 Trail Gaiters 137
Wigwam socks 67, 70, 72
Wraptor Sandal 38
Wrightsock 67
Wyoming Wear socks 75

Z

Z-Dry One socks 72
Zeasorb powder 80, 132